Asthma I

By the same author:
Arthritis – Allergy, Nutrition and the Environment

Asthma Epidemic

Dr. John Mansfield

Thorsons
An Imprint of HarperCollins*Publishers*

Thorsons
An Imprint of HarperCollins*Publishers*
77–85 Fulham Palace Road,
Hammersmith, London W6 8JB
1160 Battery Street,
San Francisco, California 94111-1213

Published by Thorsons 1997

10 9 8 7 6 5 4 3 2 1

Dr. John Mansfield asserts the moral right to
be identified as the author of this work

A catalogue record for this book
is available from the British Library

ISBN 0 7225 3600 3

Printed and bound in Great Britain by
Creative Print and Design (Wales), Ebbw Vale

To all my staff at the Burghwood Clinic,
for all the help and support they have given me
in the past 15 years.

Contents

Acknowledgements

I would especially like to thank the following physicians who have helped, guided and inspired me during the past 20 years in which I have been involved in this fascinating and stimulating approach to medicine. Many have become wonderful personal friends and others have stimulated me by their writings.

First I would like to thank Dr. David Freed of Manchester, whose thoughts and writings on this subject inspired me to write this book.

I would especially like to thank Dr. Derek Wraith for his pioneering work with food sensitivity and asthma and for agreeing to write a foreword to this book.

From the United Kingdom, I would also like to thank Dr. Ronald Finn, Dr. Stephen Davies, Dr. Michael Radcliffe, Dr. Jonathan Brostoff, Dr. Patrick Kingsley, Dr. Keith Eaton, Dr. Len McEwen and Dr. Jonathan Maberly.

From the United States, I would like to thank Prof. W. J. Rea, Dr. Joseph Miller, Dr. Sherry Rogers, Dr. W. Crook, Dr. John Trowbridge, Dr. Orion Truss, Dr. Sidney Baker, Dr. Doris Rapp and Dr. Ken Gerdes.

Drs. Richard Mackarness and Theron Randolph, who taught me so much in my early years, have unfortunately both recently died.

Finally, I would especially like to thank my Practice Manager Mrs. Jackie Bowers, for all the work she has put in typing this book.

Foreword

Identifying the cause of illness and then dealing with those causes is the highest aim of medical practice.

Asthma is a disease which has many causes, some of which have been well recognised for decades, but others, although extensively reported in the medical literature, have not as yet become as well accepted.

For much of this century it has been understood that asthma can be caused by allergy to housedust, housedust mites, moulds, animals and pollens. These allergies, for the most part, can be well demonstrated by skin prick tests, which are easy to perform and can be done quickly. These inhaled allergies, however, only account for a proportion of cases. Many cases of asthma are caused by food sensitivities which I spent much time demonstrating during my years as Visiting Consultant Chest Physician at St. Thomas' Hospital and other hospitals in London. This work has been described in detail later in this book. Food sensitivities have largely been overlooked as they cannot be satisfactorily diagnosed by skin test. They can, however, be shown using elimination diets. Chemical sensitivities can also be demonstrated by special intradermal tests or controlled challenge tests.

The huge increase in the incidence and mortality of asthma further emphasises the importance of discovering and avoiding these various causes of asthma. This is particularly important as the use of many drugs, which have an immediate and obvious short-term benefit, can in the long term probably make the underlying condition worse. There is extensive evidence for this detailed in Chapter 3.

The book throughout emphasises a holistic approach to this subject. For example, when food sensitivity is involved many other symptoms like skin disorders, fatigue, gastro-intestinal disorders, migraine and arthritis may also be present and respond at the same time to the elimination dietary procedure. Indeed, the sheer presence of many other symptoms like these, in itself, is a good indication of food sensitivity.

The author also describes how nutrients, such as magnesium and certain vitamins, play an important role in the cocktail of causative factors that lead to this condition.

Finally, and very importantly, a recent form of desensitsation is enabling physicians adequately to help most patients suffering from allergies that are unavoidable. In the past, incremental desensitization was used, but proved very ineffective for most patients and was in turn very time-consuming. It did also have some risk and the whole procedure has, as a result, been largely discontinued in the United Kingdom. In total contrast, intradermal neutralisation, which is a *totally different technique*, is usually effective within a few days, is extremely safe and well substantiated in many clinical trials.

This unique book deserves to be read by physicians who deal with asthma, and also by patients. There has never been a book which so clearly sets out all the causes of the asthma epidemic which is sweeping Western civilisation and which suggests practical and workable solutions to it.

Dr. Derek Wraith
Visiting Consultant Physician
St. Thomas' Hospital, London (retired)

1

An Introductory Overview

> At this time when mortality rates from other chronic diseases are on the decline, clinical observations in recent years have demonstrated an increase in the mortality rate from asthma in several countries.
>
> Prof. V. Serafini – Rome 1992[1]

The current management of asthma is a major disaster for both the medical profession and for people suffering from the disease.

In a recent month about 20 per cent of media medical programmes on television were related to the epidemic of asthma which is sweeping the Western world. The word 'epidemic' is not a misnomer. Most people think the term 'epidemic' is confined to infectious diseases, but in the *Concise English Dictionary* it is defined as 'a disease spreading rapidly amongst many people in one area'.

Currently in England and Wales nearly 2,000 people a year die of asthma and this figure has gone up progressively in the last 40 years, although the numbers have flattened out of late. The death rate, however, only represents the tip of the iceberg of human misery that this condition inflicts on the population. Almost three million people in the United Kingdom have asthma, and just over half of these are children. Children in classrooms queue up daily to have their asthma inhalers handed out by their teachers. Overall, over 11 per cent of children have some degree of asthma. Admission rates of children 0–4 years old have increased 15– to 20–fold in the past 35 years. The admission rates for children aged 5–14 years have increased by about four to five times. These figures relate to the United Kingdom, but similar stories are noted in other Western countries, particularly Australia, New Zealand and Finland. Economically there is also a major effect, in that about half of all patients suffering from asthma need periodically to take time off work. When patients do manage to make it to work, about 54 per cent will be working less efficiently as they experience regular night-time attacks. Parents of children suffering from asthma are generally bewildered and very ill at ease with these developments, the ever-increasing drug prescriptions and the bland assurance that little Jimmy should grow out of the problem within a few years. Many of course do not, and still have the problem right through their adult lives.

Until the 1950s asthma was rarely thought of as being a life-threatening condition. Thus the extremely eminent physician Osler wrote over 100 years ago, 'Death during an attack is almost unknown'.[2]

In 1920 the *Oxford Textbook of Medicine* wrote 'Prognosis is excellent. The sensitive type probably never dies in an attack and the non-sensitive type rarely dies in an attack.'[3] Coke[4] in 1923 wrote 'The prognosis with regard to longevity is notoriously good' and Conybeare's *Textbook of Medicine* in 1929 stated, 'It is doubtful whether death has ever been caused by uncomplicated asthma (that is asthma without emphysema).'[5]

What on earth is going on here? Here we are in 1997 in the grip of a worldwide epidemic of asthma deaths, when only a few years ago our clinical ancestors were calmly saying that it never happened. Were they all blind? Were they fools? It hardly seems likely, as death from asthma suffocation is a peculiarly horrifying spectacle not likely to pass unnoticed. These medical giants of the past were noted for the accuracy of their clinical observations, as this was the major tool of medicine in the days prior to the vast explosion of clinical tests that now dominate the medical scene. Despite this, these great physicians were so impressed by the harmlessness of asthma that they all mentioned it.

There is absolutely no doubt now that within the last four decades we have witnessed a startling increase in asthma deaths, accompanied by a huge rise in asthma prescriptions and asthma hospitalization.[6] The details of this are to be found in the next chapter.

This phenomenon troubles every doctor who sees asthma, and attempted explanations have been many. The International Consensus Report issued in 1992 by the UK National Institute of Health[7] reflects the view of most conventional drug-orientated chest physicians in that they lay the blame squarely on underdiagnosis and inappropriate treatment, which is shorthand for not enough steroids (cortisone-like drugs). But this is hardly an adequate explanation for the strange harmlessness of the condition a couple of generations ago, when treatment was primitive, steroids were unknown and some types of industrial pollution were horrific.

If we accept that for some reason asthma now is a potentially fatal condition, even though it wasn't in the recent past, then calling for earlier hospitalization and more aggressive steroid treatment appears responsible – but we still have a duty to ask why asthma has become more fatal and more widespread in occurrence. There are several disturbing factors which will probably provide the answer, and there is not much doubt in my mind that it is a combination of these factors that is at the heart of the problem. The main suspects (not in order of importance), are as follows:

Suspect 1: Outdoor Chemical Air Pollution

Certain types of outdoor air pollution have increased markedly over the past four decades, particularly nitrogen oxides from car exhausts. Nitric oxide is produced by the combustion of fuel such as petrol. After leaving the exhaust pipe it combines with oxygen in the air, forming nitrogen dioxide. I will for the rest of this book refer to nitrogen dioxide when talking of this form of pollution. However, there has been at the same time a major diminution of other types of air pollution, such as the sulphur dioxide smogs so prevalent up to about 1960. These smogs were made a thing of the past by anti-pollution legislation. However, increased pollution with nitrogen dioxide cannot be the whole story, or even the main cause of this sorry saga, as there have been major increases in the incidence of asthma even in very rural areas.

One of the most interesting studies published in relation to air pollution and asthma was authored by Dr. Jane Austin, a paediatrician at Inverness Royal Northern Infirmary.[8] In this survey she compared the prevalence of asthma amongst school-age children in the Isle of Skye, the rest of the Scottish Highlands, Aberdeen and Cardiff.

The Isle of Skye is one of the least polluted parts of the British Isles. There are no factories and very few cars. The only man-made pollution on the whole island is the smoke from some household fires, but this would be rapidly dispersed by the blustery winds so prevalent in that locality.

Despite all this, lung function tests in the children from Skye showed some degree of asthma in approximately 30 per cent. Asthma was also more common in these children than in other parts of the Highlands. Of great significance for anyone who thinks that outdoor chemical pollution is the whole story was the revelation that asthma in Skye was more common than in the city of Aberdeen, while in polluted Cardiff the rate was only 8 per cent.

The study does in fact support other, similar studies that show no constant relationship between outdoor chemical pollution and asthma. One study published in 1992 compared the incidence of asthma in Munich (in the former West Germany) and in Leipzig (in the former East Germany).[9]

Before the fall of the Berlin wall, the pollution in Leipzig was awesome. The amount of sulphur dioxide was 30 times worse than in Munich, and particulate matter in the air was 10 times worse. Despite this, asthma was found to be *more* common in Munich.

Another gas produced by traffic in cities is ozone. It mostly occurs in the summer months and is known to cause irritation of the bronchial tubes, even in otherwise healthy people. Ozone is produced by the action of sunlight on car fumes, leading to the famous photo-chemical smogs for which cities like Los Angeles are notorious. Although there was no doubt that it can make existing asthma worse, there are good grounds (as I will explain later in this chapter) to suggest that it does not play a part in initiating the whole problem.

Suspect 2: Indoor Air Pollution

Indoor air pollution has always received much less attention than outdoor air pollution, but since Dr. Theron Randolph[10] drew attention to its effects in 1962 it has received much more attention. The chemical content of houses has increased enormously over the past few decades. Most houses are now heated by gas or oil boilers which are usually situated within the living area of the house and their combustion products, even if properly maintained, spread throughout the house. Gas cookers are also extremely popular and a major source of indoor air pollution despite ventilating hoods, which do remove some of the fumes.

Gas and oil, like petrol, when burned produce nitric oxide, which then combines with oxygen to form nitrogen dioxide. This indoor type of air pollution never strikes people as a problem because it is far less obviously noxious than petrol and diesel exhaust, which looks horrible, tastes horrible, smells horrible and in every way looks the villain of the piece. However, these indoor air pollutants are usually emitted in a well-sealed house and not subject to immediate dilution by the atmosphere. Of even more importance is the fact that human exposure to these pollutants will be almost continuous, as opposed to the intermittent type of exposure that most of us have to outdoor air pollution.

Other major indoor air pollutants include:

1. Formaldehyde – found in carpets, chipboard, cavity wall insulation, foam rubber, new textiles, paper and anti-perspirants amongst many other household items.
2. Burning fat and oils in the kitchen, which produce a fine blue smoke which is well known to irritate the bronchial tubes.
3. Phenol – a gas which is given off from soft plastics.
4. Trichlorethylene – also found in carpets.
5. Toluene – the characteristic smell from gloss paint.
6. Cigarette smoke, which causes obvious asthmatic reactions in certain patients.

Thus, increasing indoor air pollution is a major suspect as it has become more prevalent in the same years that asthma has been on the rise.

Suspect 3: Is the Cure Part of the Cause?

Some of the drugs which are used to control asthma may be having a dramatically beneficial effect in the short term, but may be making the condition worse in the long term. The eminent physician, Constantine Hering, in the last century used to teach his students that the suppression of acute symptoms caused chronic symptomatology. In all fields of human endeavour, short-term beneficial solutions can have a disastrous long-term effect. In economics, for example, a reduction of the interest rate to 1 per cent will reliably cause an immediate economic boom, to be followed eventually by rampant inflation, high interest rates and a recession a year or two later.

After the upsurge in asthma-related deaths in the mid 1960s, which included well-publicized cases such as that of the Rolling Stones' Brian Jones, there was a general perception amongst the public and the medical profession that asthma inhalers were dangerous. Consumption of drugs for asthma then fell, as did the mortality rate. By the mid 1970s, however, physicians had regained their confidence with the new generation of 'safe', non-cardiotoxic bronchodilators, and prescription rates started to rise again, to be followed by death rates.[11] This fall and subsequent rise in mortality does provide a further argument against the increased pollution theory, since air pollution (at least the nitrogen dioxide from cars) was rising pretty smoothly throughout these years.[12]

At this point I can almost hear some readers thinking 'Inhalers can't be the major cause, as people wouldn't use them in the first place unless they already had asthma.' But very mild asthma is quite common in children. Over 11 per cent of children have wheezy episodes, which if left alone normally resolve by the age of 10.[13] The worry is that by calling these wheezy episodes 'asthma', which incidentally is perfectly correct, they trigger the doctor's prescribing reflex and a transient wheeze may be converted into a chronic condition that needs ever-increasing doses of inhaled drugs to keep it under control. To quote one recent Canadian review, 'we should hesitate before recommending the regular use of *any* Beta-Agonist Drug (Salbutamol, Fenoterol, etc.).'[14] Similarly, one could quote the even more provocative words of a group of New Zealand asthmologists in a paper published in *The Lancet* entitled 'Is the Cure the Cause?'[15]

By 1995 there was no doubt at all and the same group of asthmologists from the Department of Medicine at Wellington School of Medicine published a paper entitled 'The End of the New Zealand Asthma Mortality Epidemic'.[16] In New Zealand there was, if you like, a super-epidemic which was over and above the epidemic observed in most other countries. It started in 1976 and finished in approximately 1990/1991. The epidemic commenced when the long-acting beta-agonist drug, Fenoterol (Duovent/Berotec) was first introduced in 1976. The drug was used very extensively throughout New Zealand for the next 14 years, and was even available without prescription over the counter in pharmacies. I dread to think how many thousands of asthmatic patients perished in the years between 1976 and 1990. In 1990 a case control study reported that inhaled Fenoterol was associated with the epidemic.[17] The New Zealand Department of Health issued warnings about the safety of Fenoterol and restricted its availability. Within a year the death rate in New Zealand had fallen by half, and has remained on the lower level since 1990. There are more details of this somewhat horrific saga in Chapter 3, which is entitled 'Is the Cure *A* Cause?' because the cure is certainly not the *only* cause.

The reader may be interested at this point to note that Fenoterol is still used in England.

Suspect 4: The Housedust Mite and Moulds

Another factor causing an increase in asthma is undoubtedly the most famous indoor air pollutant, the housedust mite (*Dermatophagoides pyteronnisius*). It is the minute faecal particles that emanate from these creatures that cause the allergic response. Most modern homes have wall-to-wall carpeting, plenty of armchairs and cushions as well as bedding mattresses, which are the natural habitat of the housedust mite. But the modern innovation that the housedust mite most approves of is double-glazing on windows and doors, which provides total draught-proofing and considerably increases the moisture content of the home. Dust mite has to have moisture to survive; houses that are damp or are built near the sea or rivers have a higher colonization of dust mites than similar houses away from the water. Dust mites absolutely have to have moisture; in older, draughtier homes there is much less of this and dust mites often die of thirst.

While on the subject of inhaled allergies, it is perhaps appropriate to mention another source of airborne allergy that may be on the increase. I refer at this point to mould sensitivity. One of the major causes of Sick Building Syndrome has been identified as moulds. Mould spores grow in the air ducts and water tanks connected with the air conditioning units. When these units are switched off during the night and over the weekend, these spores multiply. When the units are switched on again, they spew a whole host of moulds throughout the building. Many patients I have talked to over the years have noticed that they feel worse in places that are air-conditioned.

Suspect 5: Deficiencies of Nutrients, Especially Magnesium

The factor that has probably had the least publicity up to now is the deficiency of the trace mineral magnesium. Magnesium is essential for the relaxation of smooth muscle, and the muscles in the walls of the bronchial tubes are smooth muscle. Once these muscles have gone into spasm as a result of an allergic insult, they find it difficult to relax if there is inadequate magnesium around. Recent studies in asthmatic patients have shown that giving them magnesium during an acute attack of asthma is a very effective treatment.[18] If magnesium is a good thing to have at the time of an emergency, then logic would suggest that it would be a great idea if the patient had an appropriate amount of magnesium in his or her bloodstream to prevent the attack occurring in the first place. A recent US Government survey found that the average American consumes less than 40 per cent of the recommended daily allowance (RDA) of magnesium. Dr. Mildred Seelig is the leading authority in the world on magnesium deficiency and has spent most of her life studying the subject. She has suggested that over 80 per cent of the American population is notably magnesium-deficient. Poor soils, intensive farming practices, acid rain, certain cooking practices and food processing all remove a large amount of magnesium from our food.

Apart from the effect on the smooth muscle of bronchials, magnesium deficiency has also in rats been shown to have an effect on the mast cells, which are the allergy-mediating cells. In a controlled group of rats, challenge with an allergen increased histamine, which is discharged from the mast cells only modestly in the urine and not at all in the blood. However, in rats with magnesium deficiency, urinary histamine and blood histamine levels were both greatly increased when exposed to the same allergen.[19] In other words, 'x' amount of allergic contact can produce much more reaction in rats who are magnesium deficient than those who are not. This work has not been formally repeated in human beings for obvious ethical reasons, but clinically we have observed that correcting magnesium deficiency when it has been identified by various clinical tests has produced distinct clinical improvement in our patients. We have noted that when we have sent asthmatic patients to a highly respected nutritional laboratory in London, well over half are shown to be magnesium deficient.

Suspect 6: Food Sensitivity

Food sensitivity occurs in many asthmatics. It is usually of the 'masked' variety which I will discuss in depth in Chapter 6. People can become slowly intolerant to everyday foods such as milk, wheat, corn, soy, eggs, yeast, coffee, tea and so forth, and because the consumption of these items is almost continuous the tie-up between their ingestion of these foods and their asthma is in no way obvious. Severe reactions to foods eaten occasionally, such as peanuts, are very obvious and are well understood, but they are far less common than the 'masked' variety. Patients who are clearly reacting to obvious inhalant allergens are labelled as suffering from 'Extrinsic asthma'. When the asthma appears not to be related to such allergies, it is labelled 'Intrinsic asthma', which is really another word for 'Don't Know'. Most of those who are labelled with 'Intrinsic asthma' are in fact suffering from food intolerance or Candida hypersensitivity (*see below*). But, as few asthma sufferers are ever put through an elimination dietary procedure, most patients and their physicians are unaware of the cause of their problems. Dr. Derek Wraith, who has now retired from his position as Chest Physician at St. Thomas' Hospital in London, has contributed more than anyone to documenting the relationship of food sensitivity to asthma. His findings were published in the tome *Food Allergy and Intolerance*,[20] and will feature extensively in Chapter 6.

Food intolerance is thought to be caused in part by highly repetitive consumption of certain foods that are major parts of our diet, such as grains, milk, eggs, sugar, yeast, etc. Certainly many patients who are sensitive to foods have highly repetitive diets, but whether this is on the increase or not is difficult to say. The chemical adulteration of food with pesticides, insecticides, sulphur dioxide, azodyes, anti-staling agents, flavouring agents, etc. is certainly on the increase, and these chemicals have been implicated by allergists in specific individuals.

Suspect 7: Candida Hypersensitivity

I devote a whole chapter in the latter part of this book to this interesting subject. Candida albicans is the medical name for thrush. Work originating in the US has suggested that a hypersensitivity to this organism, which is a universal occupant of the human gut, may be behind a small but significant number of cases of asthma. Certainly we have observed a number of people with asthma who have responded excellently to a regime of anti-fungal drugs such as Nystatin, Amphotericin and Diflucan, combined with a diet low in sugar and yeast products. There are theoretical grounds for believing that this organism is more prevalent in the human gut nowadays than it was 60 years ago. Factors that encourage its growth are sugar, antibiotics and the contraceptive pill. The consumption of sugar has risen spectacularly in the last 90 years, from about 2 pounds per person per year to 144 pounds per person per year. Antibiotics were unknown until 1940, and are now used extensively both to treat human beings and to deal with the animals which we later consume. The contraceptive pill was unknown until the 1950s and is now used extensively over very long periods of time. Many women never experience vaginal thrush until they have been on the contraceptive pill.

Countless people observe that they have diarrhoea after treatment with antibiotics. The antibiotics kill beneficial bacteria as well as the harmful ones. The beneficial bacteria includes the *Lactobacillus acidophilus*. This organism acts in competition with the yeast organism Candida albicans, which can then multiply rapidly if the Lactobacillus is suppressed. There is now quite a lot of published evidence that this yeast is implicated in certain selected cases of asthma; I will go into more detail in Chapter 8.

We thus have our seven suspects all lined up. Clearly there is not just one villain and clearly the problem can be divided into '**What causes the problem in the first instance?**' and then '**What perpetuates it?**'

Let us now look primarily as to what may be causing the problem in the first place. Clearly, the increased incidence of asthma has been so dramatic in the last 40 years that genetic change can be discounted. Genes spread very slowly – a mutant gene could not possibly spread so rapidly as to cause this sort of increase within two generations. Almost certainly at the root of the problem is a phenomenon called 'Tolerance Induction'. We all have an immune system which is similar to a defensive army, and this protects us from a huge range of insults which our environment is inclined to throw at us. These include bacteria, viruses, fungii, yeasts, toxins and allergens.

The prime function of the immune system is to distinguish between invaders that may be harmful from those that are harmless. Thus the immune system should act effectively against microbes which may cause disease, but not react against harmless items such as pollen, dust, dust mite and food molecules.

The act of learning to distinguish and shrug off items that are harmless is called '**Tolerance Induction**'. This process occurs when we first as a baby meet a new allergen.

In mice and rats it has been shown that an antigen (an item that is a potential allergen) if inhaled automatically induces tolerance and prevents any production of the antibody Immunoglobulin E (IgE for short). It works through the good offices of some very special cells called T-suppressor cells, but unfortunately this system is not very well established in newborn rats or mice. Hence at this time in their lives they can be relatively easily sensitized by an inhaled antigen. This may well explain why, for example, human beings are more likely to develop hayfever if they are born just before the hayfever season.

Of enormous importance is the fact that it has been shown that, even in adult rats and mice, **the inhalation of certain chemicals can interfere with their 'induction of tolerance'**. High on the list of chemicals that can interfere in this way is the gas nitrogen dioxide, which as I have already described is not only present in car exhaust fumes but is also spewed out from gas cookers and gas and oil boilers. These indoor air pollutants are normally discharged into hermetically-sealed homes, where they remain for some time. Thus if an animal inhales a fair amount of nitrogen dioxide, it can irritate the nose and the adjacent upper respiratory system. If this animal then inhales an antigen like housedust mite to which it has never previously been exposed, it will not become tolerant in the normal course of events.

Sulphur dioxide, which was such a major pollutant earlier this century, has also been shown in experimental animals to prevent Tolerance Induction, but most sulphur dioxide was always encountered outside the house and was therefore subject to dispersal in the atmosphere. Ozone, for its part, has been shown *not* to interfere with Tolerance Induction.

These studies on Tolerance Induction were performed on mice and rats; whether the same effect occurs in human beings is not known for sure. However, scientists think that it is almost certain that it does, as it is such a fundamental biological mechanism.

Thus:

1. The housedust mite is by far the most common single cause of asthma in the UK. In countries more than 600 miles nearer the equator, dust mites are rare.
2. It thrives in the humidity occurring in hermetically-sealed double-glazed homes.
3. Gas and oil utilities are frequently used in these same homes and produce nitrogen dioxide, which is thus also retained.
4. Of very distinct significance in this respect was a study published in the *American Journal of Epidemiology*.[21] This was a case control study amongst children aged 3 or 4 years old, diagnosed for the first time with asthma. In these children there was a striking association between the incidence of asthma and nitrogen dioxide exposure as

measured with a personal badge over a period of 24 hours. I will expand on this later in Chapter 7 on chemical sensitivity, but we can now begin to see a scenario which fits with the known facts concerning the increased incidence of asthma.

It would appear the **concurrent inhalation of indoor chemical pollutants and biological inhaled allergens such as dust, dust mite, feathers, moulds and animal fur in modern hermetically-sealed homes is very likely to be the reason why most asthma starts in the first place.** This concept would mainly fit the development of what many asthma specialists refer to as Extrinsic Asthma. This refers to asthma patients who have a history suggestive of dust mite and mould sensitivity backed up by positive skin prick tests. Intrinsic Asthma is another story, which we will discuss later.

I hope I have now managed to lay to rest the concept that outdoor air pollution is the main problem. Apart from being wrong, this idea tends to lead to an air of defeatism in regard to helping asthma, as it is highly unlikely, even with the introduction of catalytic convertors, that a major change will occur in outdoor chemical pollution within the next 20 years. The realization that even if we reduced air pollution to the levels seen of the Isle of Skye we would still have a massive problem, directs our attention towards factors which will be much easier to manipulate.

I hope the reader will find hope and inspiration in the rest of this book for dealing with this problem positively. The general message is that it is about time we relied less on drugs and got down seriously to dealing with the basic causes of asthma. There are some drugs that seem to be both helpful and harmless, and these are fine although rarely will they be the whole answer. What we can do with what we already know is pretty extensive.

We can, for example,

1. take measures to minimize our contact with dust, dust mites, moulds and animals whenever they appear to be the problem.
2. desensitize people who have inhaled allergies quickly, efficiently and safely with a technique known as neutralization. This technique is totally different from the old-fashioned incremental densensitization, which was generally speaking very unsuccessful and had some risks. Neutralization, in contrast, is very successful, usually within a week or two, employs very low doses of allergens, which actually have a negative skin reaction, and enables most people

within 12 days to inhale allergens without producing an asthmatic reaction.

3. identify chemical sensitivity by skin test and other similar techniques.

4. control most forms of indoor air pollution and desensitize patients to chemicals that are unavoidable.

5. enhance, with nutritional supplementation, the ability of our enzyme systems to detoxify chemicals and render them harmless.

6. sort out food sensitivity with elimination diets or intradermal provocative skin testing, in patients where this appears to be a problem. It is also possible to densensitize people to foods which have been identified as problems during the course of an elimination diet.

7. treat the candida/yeast problem using anti-fungal medications and sugar-free/yeast-free diets when appropriate.

8. test accurately for both magnesium and all the other nutrients involved in our detoxification system. This helps us to correct these abnormalities and enable patients to cope with chemicals in their environment, either indoor or outdoor.

Many physicians are now finding that with this type of approach we can enable many asthma sufferers to leave their medications at home.

What is Asthma and How Common Is It?

The symptoms associated with bronchial asthma are caused by a narrowing of both the bronchii (the large tubes) and the bronchioles (the small tubes) in the lungs. This narrowing is caused by the contraction of the smooth muscle within the walls of these tubes, and by viscid secretions that obstruct the tubes.

Asthma is the single most common chronic disease of childhood, affecting about 11 per cent of all school children. About 80 per cent of children with asthma have their first attack before the age of five, and approximately half of them will stop having the problem by the time they become adults.

The most obvious symptoms of this condition are recurrent cough, wheezing or shortness of breath, possibly occurring predominantly during the night or after exercise.

The condition with which asthma is most frequently confused is an acute bronchial infection or bronchitis. In both, the doctor can hear a rhonchi (wheezing) in the chest with the help of a stethoscope. Alternatively these noises can be heard by the simple expedient of placing an ear against the chest wall. Rapid relief of symptoms by the use of a bronchodilator (an anti-asthma drug that relaxes smooth muscles in the bronchial tubes) favours the diagnosis of asthma, as these drugs work very poorly when, as in bronchitis, the wheeze is caused by an infection. If the symptoms are transient and intermittent it is more likely to be asthma than bronchitis. In a patient suffering from bronchitis the symptoms tend to be absent for months at a time and then become markedly apparent for several days or a week or so. Bronchitis is also often associated with the production of infected sputum.

Viral infections can precipitate asthma. If a virus alone is involved in the process, antibiotics are of no value.

The Increase in the Incidence of Asthma and the Mortality of Asthma

This increase is both very extensive, very well documented and is accepted as valid by all the leading authorities on this subject. At one time a few voices did suggest that the increase was at least partly due to changes in diagnostic fashion amongst doctors. Perhaps 30 years ago a transient wheeze might have been more likely to be labelled bronchitis and is now more likely to be termed asthma. This might have slightly 'skewed' the statistics, but it is agreed that this could have had only a small effect on the numbers.

Apart from all the statistical evidence that followed, school teachers who have taught in schools since the 1960s know that, whereas in those years perhaps one child per class carried an asthma inhaler, it is nowadays common for about a fifth of the class to queue up for their inhalers at lunchtime. This is a peculiarly sick phenomenon, if one thinks about it, for a supposedly advanced civilized society with a supposedly sophisticated medical service.

Furthermore, there is no doubt at all that in the past few years, around 2,000 people have been dying each year of asthma in England and Wales. Between 1988 and 1992 the number was over 2,000 but it has dropped slightly to just under 2,000 in the last couple of years.

As mentioned in the introductory chapter, until the 1950s asthma was very rarely regarded as life-threatening and the standard textbooks of medicine, such as the *Oxford Textbook of Medicine* and *Conybeare's Textbook of Medicine*, emphasized the benignity of the condition in regard to mortality. This was despite the horrific pollution brought about by the Industrial Revolution beginning in the mid-19th century.

Studying the Increase in Asthma since 1960

A number of studies have been reported covering different periods of time in the last 45 years. The UK Asthma Task Force, for example, recently disclosed that the number of people with asthma has doubled even in the last 10 years. During that time hospital admissions have trebled for all victims; for young children they have risen five-fold.

However, the increase had been well underway long before the last 10 years. In the UK's 'National Study of Health and Growth 1973–86,'[1] approximately 30,000 children were studied. The conclusion was that there was a true increase in the incidence of asthma which was not accounted for by changes in diagnostic fashion. Perhaps one picture can convey more than a thousand statistics: Figure 1 shows the trend of hospital admissions for children in the period from 1958 to 1986. This study represented an increase of 1,300 per cent in the 0–4 age group and 600 per cent in the 5–14 age group.

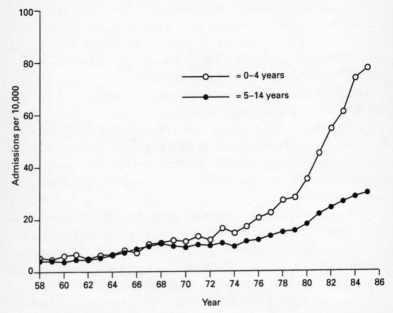

Figure 1 Trends in hospital admissions for asthma in England and Wales: 1958–85, for ages 0–4 and 5–14 years (sexes combined)

In a separate study,[2] limited to England's south-west Thames region and covering the years 1970–85, the conclusion showed a smaller but still very distinct increase. The timespan for this study was only 15 years as opposed to 28 years for the National Study, but it still showed an increase of 186 per cent in the 0–4 age group, and 56 per cent in the 5–14 age group.

A major study in South Wales compared the results of a survey performed in 1973 with an identical one performed in 1988.[3] Twelve-year-old children were surveyed within a specifically defined area of South Wales. Questionnaires and peak expiratory flow rates were completed for 965 children. All the peak expiratory flow rates were then repeated after an exercise provocation test. The 1973 survey was repeated in 1985, again with twelve-year-old children and identical methodology. The prevalence of wheeze at any time had increased from 17 to 22 per cent of these children. Asthma at any time had increased from 6 to 12 per cent, and current asthma had increased from 4 to 9 per cent. In other words, there was roughly a doubling of the rate of asthma in that particular 15-year timespan.

Another study[4] compared not only asthma but also hayfever in patients who came to consult their doctors in England and Wales, in 1970/71 and 1981/82. Within these years the prevalence of asthma in men increased from 11.6 to 20.5 people consulting per thousand of the population, and women in 8.8 to 15.9 people consulting per thousand population. Similar increases were noted in the data compiled from the 19 health centres contributing to both surveys.

Some of the most troubling news has come from Australia, where Robertson and his colleagues compared the prevalence of asthma in Melbourne school children over a period of 26 years. The most incredible statistic in this study showed that, whereas in 1964 the prevalence of a history of asthma in 7-year-old children was 19.1 per cent, by 1990 the prevalence was 46 per cent. This was an increase in these 26 years of 141 per cent. It is almost unbelievable that nearly one half of Melbourne school children have a history of asthma. Over and above that, Australia has the second-highest reported mortality from asthma in the world, and in the years between 1980 and 1990 the mortality in the 0–19 age group increased by 50 per cent.

These findings were confirmed by Dr. Peat and his colleagues, who studied children in the 8–10 age group in two separate country towns in Australia's New South Wales region.[5] This study was particularly important as it reported objective measurements, whereas the Melbourne study[6] was based on responses to a questionnaire. This study showed that airway hyper-responsiveness increased by somewhere between 1.4 and two-fold within 10 years. Although airway hyper-responsiveness is not totally correlated with asthma, this marked increase is objective evidence of a very serious problem at work here.

Very similar high rates of asthma were seen when virtually identical questionnaires were used in Fiji[7] and Las Serena,[8] a non-polluted town in northern Chile.

In Germany the rates are much lower, at figures somewhere between 4 and 6 per cent; in Switzerland, the overall rate of asthma hovers around 7 per cent.

In New Zealand there was between 1976 and 1991 perhaps the worst epidemic of asthma mortality seen anywhere in the world,[9] but this appears to have been caused by a long-acting bronchodilator drug which was used very extensively in that country. Since its withdrawal the rate has dropped dramatically (the whole saga is explored in Chapter 3). We end this discourse on the increase in asthma with a study from Finland,[10] examining the prevalence of asthma in Finnish young men between 1926 and 1989. These figures were obtained at the time of medical examination prior to military conscription. All of these figures were noted at the time of this initial medical examination. The first and highest graph shown in Figure 2 gives the percentage of men with the diagnosis of asthma at or before call-up for medical examination (the line with small square boxes in it). The second line, marked with black dots, represents the percentage of men exempted at call-up for military service by virtue of disabling asthma. The third line, marked with

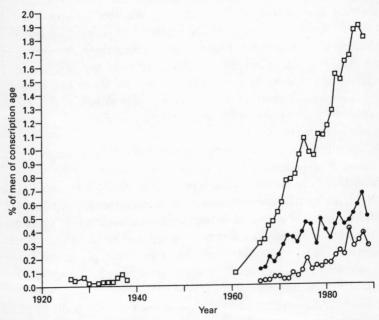

Figure 2 Prevalence of asthma in Finnish young men during 1926–89 expressed as a percentage of male candidates for military conscription with diagnosis of asthma at or before call up medical examination (☐), percentage of men exempted at call up for military service by virtue of disabling asthma (●), and percentage of conscripts discharged during course of military service because of asthma (○)

circles, delineates the percentage of conscripts discharged during the course of military service because of asthma.

Figure 2 exemplifies very well that the early 1960s were the take-off point for the major increases in asthma seen in very many Western countries.

The Cost of Asthma

Asthma affects between 2.5 and 3 million people in the UK alone. Over 61,000 British asthma sufferers were asked to report the frequency of their symptoms. The results are shown in Figure 3.

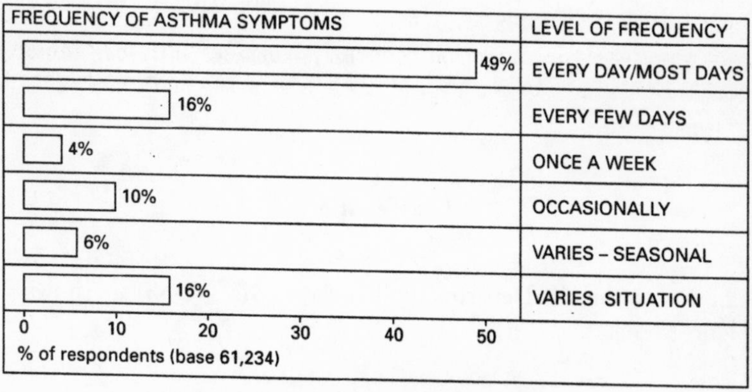

FREQUENCY OF ASTHMA SYMPTOMS	LEVEL OF FREQUENCY
49%	EVERY DAY/MOST DAYS
16%	EVERY FEW DAYS
4%	ONCE A WEEK
10%	OCCASIONALLY
6%	VARIES – SEASONAL
16%	VARIES SITUATION

0   10   20   30   40   50
% of respondents (base 61,234)

Figure 3   Frequency of asthma symptoms

In 1992 the cost of the condition to Britain's National Health Service (NHS) were reported, although as these figures were compiled in1988, the figures would by now be distinctly higher. Doctors' (GPs') costs and hospital costs are shown in Figure 4.

GP COSTS	
4.6 million consultations	£33,000,000
27 million prescriptions	£228,000,000
SUB-TOTAL	£261,000,000

HOSPITAL COSTS	
575,000 in-patient bed days	£73,100,000
41,000 out-patient referrals plus 120,000 out-patient attendances	£10,300,000[1]
SUB-TOTAL	£83,400,000

NOTES TO THE ACCOUNTS:
This is a conservative estimate.
If allowance is made for inflation
since 1988, when the figures
were compiled, the estimate
can be revised upwards to
around £400million!

NHS TOTAL COSTS per year (rounded up)	**£345,000,000**

Figure 4 GP costs

The cost to the UK Department of Social Services (DSS) are shown in Figure 5.

DSS COSTS	
Sickness benefit 0.8 million days plus invalidity benefit 4.9 million days.	£60,000,000
TOTAL COST TO THE DSS per year	**£60,000,000**

Figure 5 Department of Social Security costs

Therefore, allowing for a little inflation between 1988 and 1992, the cost to the UK taxpayer for the National Health Service is as shown in Figure 6.

DESCRIPTION	COST	
For: All costs relating to ASTHMA including:		
– NHS costs (GP and Hospital)	£400,000,000	00
– DSS costs (sickness and invalidity benefit)	£60,000,000	00
TOTAL TO PAY	£460,000,000	00

Figure 6   Costs to the UK taxpayer

Over and above this there are major costs to the national economy in terms of working days lost (see Figure 7).

In Britain 7.1 million working days are lost each year with a loss of potential productivity estimated at	£342,000,000
TOTAL COST per year	**£342,000,000**

Figure 7   Costs to the UK economy

If we add this £342 million to the £460 million cost to the National Health Service, the figure comes to over £800 million loss to the economy in general. A major programme of dealing with asthma in terms of cause and effect would, apart from relieving untold misery, lead to a huge economic benefit for the UK as a whole, as it would for any country willing to embark on such a programme.

Is the Cure a Cause?

The short answer to this question is an unequivocal *Yes*. The single most dramatic piece of evidence relates to the huge drop in the mortality rate in New Zealand in 1990 when the use of the long acting beta-agonist drug Fenoterol (Berotec/Duovent) became highly restricted. The death rate from asthma dropped by approximately one-half in the year 1990–91.[1]

Before I go into the extensive evidence that most asthma drugs are dangerous, allow me to say that not all of them are. As far as we know the best totally harmless drugs are the mast cell stabilizers, of which the best known are Intal (sodium cromoglycate) and Tilade (sodium nedocromil). Both of these work by tackling the allergic reaction at an early stage by making the mast cells in the lining of the bronchii more stable. If these cells are more stable they are less likely to liberate their chemicals, histamine and leucotrines, in response to an allergic challenge: hence asthma is less likely to result.

However, these drugs need to get to the mast cells before the allergen and so these medications need to be taken regularly. Normally the worst effect they can have is to make the patient sneeze, or to irritate the throat and produce a cough. Very rarely, they have brought on an asthma attack.

Intal and Tilade work well with some patients who have purely inhaled allergies, but appear useless when food sensitivity is the main cause of the problem. Poor response to mast cell stabilizers can in fact be a good indicator of food sensitivity. These drugs are safe because when they do work they stop the reaction before it even starts and do not suppress wheezing. Neither is of any use once an attack has started, however.

In contrast, the group of drugs that are most worrying are the beta 2 agonists. These drugs are currently the most commonly employed medication once an attack is underway. The use of effective drugs for the symptomatic treatment of asthma has had an extremely checkered past; as early as 1948 Benson & Pearlman[2] calculated that the use of adrenalin sprays had resulted in a five-fold increase in asthma mortality. Subsequent mortality peaks followed the introduction of Isoprenaline, and again after the introduction of high dosage Isoprenaline. By the mid-1960s there was a general perception amongst the public and the medical profession that asthma inhalers were dangerous; as a result prescriptions fell, as did the mortality rate. In the mid-1970s physicians had regained their confidence with the new generation of bronchodilators, which had no effect on the heart and were initially thought of as safe. Prescription rates began to rise again, to be followed by an increase in death rates.

Soon it was becoming clear that these new, more selective beta 2 agonists had a 'down side' to them. In the original paper by Benson & Pearlman concerning the dangers of adrenaline it had been noted that some of the excessive mortality appeared to be in patients who took the adrenaline by use of a nebulizer, which in 1948 was available over the counter in the US. Similarly, some of the excess mortality in the New Zealand epidemic appeared to be related to the use of Fenoterol in conjunction with pressurized nebulizers. Much higher doses of the drug are inhaled with nebulizers as opposed to the doses attained with metered dose inhalers or dry powder aerosols.

The case against Fenoterol (sold as Berotec or Duovent) is pretty well incontrovertible. The New Zealand 'super-epidemic' commenced when Fenoterol was introduced in 1976. There was then a very high death rate for the next 13 years. In mid-1989 the first Fenoterol case study was published.[3] There were major safety worries, and the use of the drug, which had been available even without prescription, was severely restricted. The market share of Fenoterol fell sharply, accompanied by a major fall in death rate within even six months. There was a further fall in the next six months, by which time the mortality rate for asthma in New Zealand had been reduced by one-half.

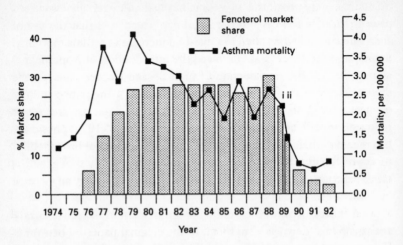

Figure 8 Inhaled fenoterol market share and annual asthma mortality in persons aged 5–34 years. The data for 1989 are divided into two 6-month periods because the first Department of Health warnings about the safety of fenoterol were issued in mid-1989.

Figure 8 in itself depicts extremely compelling evidence, but the fact that the epidemic in New Zealand has remained at this much lower level from 1991 to the present day is even more impressive.

The Wellington Asthma Research Group concluded their summary in the paper entitled 'The End of the New Zealand Asthma Mortality Epidemic'[4] with the words 'The New Zealand time trends in asthma death are consistent with Fenoterol being the main cause of the New Zealand asthma mortality epidemic and are inconsistent with a significant role for other suggestive causes.'

Somewhat incredibly, Fenoterol is still very widely prescribed in the UK.

The other widely used long-acting beta-agonist is Salmeterol (trade name Serevent). In July 1995 Dr. B. Lipworth of the University of Dundee produced a paper in *The Lancet* entitled 'Bronchodilator Subsensitivity to Salbutamol after twice daily Salmeterol in Asthma Patients'.[5] Patients were randomized to receive Salmeterol 50 ug twice daily for a placebo for 4 weeks in a double-blind cross-over fashion. It was found that the patients pre-treated with Salmeterol had a reduced response to Salbutamol, in terms of both forced expiratory volume and peak expiratory flow rates, than those treated with placebo. The reduction in response equated with a 2½- to 4-fold greater dosage of Salbutamol being required to produce the same benefit as found in the placebo group.

In other words, the use of the long-acting beta 2 agonist Salmeterol meant one had to use a much higher dosage of the short-acting beta agonist Salbutamol to achieve the same result. In 1993 a Canadian study demonstrated worrying results even with the shorter-acting beta 2 agonists.[6] After just two weeks' use of regular Salbutamol there was an increased reaction of the airways to the same amount of allergen. In the summary it was stated that the effect of inhaled beta agonists provided further evidence to support the detrimental effects of using them regularly.

Another study of beta 2 agonists conducted by a variety of medical schools in the US and Canada, including Montreal General Hospital and Yale University,[7] showed that the use of beta agonists administered by a metered dose inhaler (specifically Salbutamol and Fenoterol) was associated with an increased risk of death or near-death.

Several other studies have shown that regular inhalation of beta 2 agonists causes 'hyper-responsiveness'—that is, excessive constriction of the bronchii.[8] There are a lot of other similar studies all coming to the same sort of conclusion, but I won't go on as I do not wish to belabour this point.

We now come to the steroids (or cortisone-like drugs). Many patients have an unholy fear of these medications, with some justification. Because of the bad news about the beta 2 agonists, many doctors are now turning to steroids as their first port of call. However, steroids, even of the inhaled variety, are still dangerous. At one time there had been a concensus of opinion that beclomethasone diproprionate (Becotide/Becodisks/Bentide, etc.) in a dosage of 400–800 ug daily was an appropriate dosage for three- to five-year-old children. However, a group of paediatric consultants from various hospitals in England wrote to *The Lancet* in December 1991 to point out various studies where these doses were the equivalent of 20–40 mg Prednisolone in causing suppression of the adrenal and pituitary glands. This dosage also produced significant growth retardation in the group of children studied. Inhaled steroids have also caused symptoms characteristic of Cushing's syndrome—that is, obesity, moon-face, thinning skin and stretch marks.

A study from Cardiff,[9] for example, published in the *British Medical Journal* set out specifically to measure skin thickness and evidence of purpura (a skin rash). They found that the high-dose inhaled corticosteroid treatment group had significantly thinner skin at all three sites observed. Differences between the placebo group and a low-dose inhaled steroid group were only minor. Ten out of 21 patients in the high-dose inhaled steroid group showed evidence of purpura.

Another risk is that otherwise benign infections can become much more serious or even life-threatening in children on drugs such as steroids which suppress the immune system. The American Food & Drug Administration has asked the manufacturers of *all* steroids to add the following warning to the drug's packaging: *Children who are on immune-suppressant drugs are more susceptible to infection than healthy children. Chicken pox and measles for example can have a more serious or even fatal course in children on immune-suppressive drugs.*

In adults, some studies have shown that even low doses of inhaled beclomethasone (400 ug per day) reduced bone formation.[10] All the steroids also cause recurrent oral thrush in the mouth of many people who use them, sometimes associated with a loss of voice.

This all brings us back to the teaching of Constantine Hering, one of the giants of medicine in the 19th century. He taught his students that the suppression of acute symptoms causes chronic symptoms.

Asthma is an immunologic process that leads to inflammation. That is to say that allergy is one of the body's natural defence mechanisms, and therefore according to this line of thought asthma itself must be protective in some way against some insult. *Mother nature did not put smooth muscle into our bronchial tubes just to make trouble*. There is a clear need to differentiate in our thinking between symptoms that represent a bodily defence mechanism and symptoms that are brought about by straightforward poisoning.

When the bronchial airways are narrowed in asthma, most attention is focused on the sensation of breathlessness and the effort required to breathe. However, although the amount of air passing through the bronchii may be reduced, its velocity and turbulence are increased,[11] giving rise to a 'scouring' action that encourages the mucus to become detached from the inner wall of the bronchials and forced upwards towards the throat. Within this mucus could be the inhaled allergens and chemicals; this mechanism would therefore have a cleansing effect on the lung. This cleaning mechanism would also be seriously compromised by any drug that permitted the secretion of mucus but prevented it from being carried away. Beta 2 agonists inhibit the bronchii constriction that initiates this scouring action and so would be expected to result in this problem. Steroids wouldn't cause this problem in that they suppress inflammation. However, steroids are problematic in all sorts of other ways, as has been described.

To reiterate some remarks in the introductory chapter, the crux of the matter is that approximately 11 per cent of all children have very mild wheezy episodes which will often resolve spontaneously by the time the child is 10 years old. By labelling these wheezy episodes asthma, which is not incorrect, they trigger the well-intentioned doctor to prescribe inhalers which will give instant and spectacular relief. However, this may cause a benign transient wheeze to convert into a chronic condition needing ever-increasing drugs to keep it under control.

To see a child wheezing is a very unpleasant experience for a parent, and it is not being suggested that Ventolin or other similar inhalers should be withheld in these circumstances. What *is* being suggested is:

1. Long-acting beta agonists should be avoided if at all possible.
2. Short-acting beta agonists should be used only when absolutely necessary, and should *not* be used in any sort of regular preventive role.
3. A vigorous search should be made to discover the cause of the individual's asthma and to deal with or reduce the exposure to such causes so that far less reliance is placed on drugs.

Four People with Asthma

I have chosen four cases of asthma managed from the viewpoint of allergy, environmental, and nutritional medicine to give the reader a flavour of how these problems can be approached. These patients are all 'run of the mill', everyday type patients, but each illustrates the diversity of factors which can lead to the condition we know as asthma. The reader will not, at this stage of the book, understand all the implications, for example of chemical sensitivity and the candida hyper-sensitivity problem; perhaps this chapter will be worth re-reading after the chapters discussing these particular factors have been read.

The first case illustrates a problem of biological inhalant allergy involving reactions to dust, dust mite and various summer pollens. This case is typical of over 40 per cent of the cases we see and they are, generally speaking, very easy to deal with. Many of these patients only require a consultation early on in the day, followed by several hours of skin testing, in turn followed by a course of neutralizing injections (self-administered).

The second case demonstrates the role that food sensitivity can play in this condition and how it can be rectified by an elimination diet.

The third case is a little more complicated, showing asthma resulting from both food *and* inhaled allergies.

The fourth case was highly complex and took many months of investigation before a really satisfactory result was obtained. However, there was considerable improvement in the symptomatology within a few weeks. This case demonstrated a complex mixture of food, inhalant and chemical sensitivities, complicated by the candida hyper-sensitivity problem and nutritional deficiencies.

1. Master G.B. (aged 7)

This boy was referred by his doctor to my clinic in May 1995. He suffered from both asthma and hayfever. The hayfever symptomatology largely affected his eyes and nose. The asthma would occur at any time throughout the year, but was significantly worse between the months of April and August, suggesting that summer pollens were playing a part in the asthma as well as his hayfever. As his symptoms would disappear if he was taken by his parents to the Mediterranean area, we were fairly certain that his problems were caused entirely by inhaled allergens such as pollens, dust and dust mite.

On skin testing, using the intradermal provocation neutralization test, he was found to be very sensitive to both house dust and dust mite, and quite sensitive to tree pollens, weeds, flowers and grass pollens. There were also reactions to hay and what is known as mixed threshings. Prior to attending the clinic he had been taking Triludan (2 daily), 4 puffs of Intal daily, Salbutamol (2 puffs at night) and Opticrom eye drops when needed.

He started taking his neutralizing injections, and within two weeks of doing this he was able to discontinue all his other medications. A sweat test at the Biolab Medical Unit revealed a zinc deficiency, but no magnesium deficiency. Three months later on follow-up his mother reported that he was very well indeed and was using no medication at all other than the neutralization treatment.

A case such as this normally requires skin testing for about 5 hours by a trained nurse. This day of medical attention can stop asthma in its tracks. After about one year of neutralizing injections, taken on alternate days, the patient is usually 'cured' in that he has no symptoms, is taking no medication and has managed to stop using his neutralizing injections. Usually the worst that can happen in these patients is that the 'turn-off levels' can change after a few months, which might lead to a slight recurrence of symptoms. Two or three hours of retesting can usually resolve this problem immediately and set the patient back on course.

2. Mrs. S.J. (aged 60)

This woman first consulted me in 1991. She had asthma for which she was taking Becotide inhalers twice a day and Ventolin when she needed it, which was usually two or three times each day. Over and above this she was badly overweight at 16 stone (224 lb). She had considerable fatigue, osteo-arthritis of her knees, bloating and wind.

There was no evidence of inhalant sensitivity in her case, but there was a great deal that suggested food sensitivity. Accordingly we put her on a low-risk allergy diet of 17 foods. After six days on this diet her asthma had totally disappeared, as had her headaches, fatigue, depression and food cravings. In addition, in this six days she lost nine pounds in weight. When she reintroduced other foods back into her diet, she showed marked reactions to wheat, corn, soy and tomatoes. She later took neutralizing injections to enable her to eat these foods without reaction. Except when she would eat these four foods, her asthma totally disappeared and her weight reduced spectacularly. She also had a little bit of the candida hypersensitivity problem; treating that produced further improvement in her other symptomatology.

3. Mrs. R.W. (aged 82)

There is a condition referred to as 'late onset asthma', and in this woman's case it started when she was 80 years old and she consulted me when she was 82! She was taking Pulmicort and Bricanyl inhalers for her problem and was also consuming Volterol Retard anti-inflammatory drugs for her arthritis, present in her knees, back and neck. She had a history of hayfever and she knew that contact with dust would make her sneeze and cough. Her history also revealed some possibility of chemical sensitivity, in that contact with car fumes and similar chemicals would make her feel quite sick. I felt that we should investigate biological inhalant allergy as well as food and chemical sensitivities. On skin testing she had moderate reactions to house dust and dust mite and lesser reactions to moulds, Alternaria, Cephalosporium, Cladosporium and Aspergillae. There were also reactions to gas and formaldehyde. Sweat tests and blood tests showed deficiencies of magnesium, zinc and chromium, as well as a major deficiency of certain essential fatty acids.

There was some improvement in her asthma after she started taking the neutralizing injections for the inhaled allergies, but there was a much greater improvement after seven days on a 17-safe foods diet. She, incidentally, on this diet, also lost her indigestion, and her arthritis was 65 per cent improved by her own estimation. Reintroducing foods back into her diet, while still continuing to take her inhalant neutralizing injections, she showed adverse reactions to soy, wheat, corn, rye, beet sugar, dates and monosodium glutamate.

On skin testing she had good skin responses to the adverse foods and started taking neutralizing injections to enable her to eat these foods. She also took supplements to correct the trace mineral and essential fatty acids deficiencies. When I saw her three months later she looked about 10 years younger, had no asthma, felt very well and even had a 70 per cent improvement in her arthritis, and all this while taking absolutely no medication at all

4. Mrs. Y.S. (aged 53)

This woman had had asthma since the age of 25, and for most of that time it had been quite severe. In addition to the asthma, she looked very ill and toxic. She told me that she suffered from frequent severe sore throats, painful joints, very severe migraines and very bad mental confusion and fatigue. The migraines occurred at least once every week and sometimes two or three times.

Thus, although she had severe asthma it was only part of her overall problem, and when all her symptoms were added up they indicated a very severely ill woman.

As emphasized in other parts of this book, we do not consider asthma in isolation from other medical complaints, and by getting at the underlying allergic and nutritional problems and correcting them, all sorts of good things can then start to happen. Before she had even consulted us, she had observed that her joint pains improved markedly on a low-risk food allergy diet.

In 1989, she had had a major exposure to a wide range of perfumes and had since noted that relatively minor exposure would cause her to feel disorientated and unable to function mentally. Other chemical exposure, such as to petrol, diesel, disinfectants and paint would produce symptoms if she inhaled them, but far and away her worst problem was with cigarette smoke, which could be guaranteed to initiate a major attack of asthma. Thus, already there were a number of clues that she had both food and chemical sensitivities. Over and above these, she had a lot of 'candida hypersensitivity-like' symptomatology, such as wind, bloating, constipation alternating with diarrhoea, poor memory and concentration, recurring cystitis and a lot of premenstrual symptomatology.

We elected to put her on an Anti-Candida diet and to give her anti-fungals, to skin test her and desensitize her to her food allergens, and to use the same technique for dealing with the chemical sensitivities. Taking neutralization therapy for foods and chemicals and dealing with the candida problem led to her asthma disappearing entirely within a few months. By this time the migraines were only occurring as a result of an occasional major exposure to perfumes.

In Chapter 7 I explain how these sensitivities are often second to nutritional deficiencies. Through the Biolab Medical Unit in London we found that this woman was deficient in the minerals zinc, chromium and, very significantly, molybdenum, all of which are important in the detoxification of chemicals. After giving her supplements of these minerals and an amino acid complex called Glutathione Complex there was a further improvement in her chemical sensitivity.

In another couple of months she had totally lost her asthma, her chemical sensitivity was vastly improved, there were no migraines and her feelings of malaise, toxicity and mental confusion had all gone. She was amazed that her memory had returned and she became much less clumsy, she could walk fast and move her tongue around her mouth quite fast for the first time in many years. On a follow-up a few months later, she informed me that she had remained symptom-free.

I could have put many hundreds of case histories similar to these in this book, but I feel that these suffice to indicate the many factors that can lie at the heart of asthma symptoms.

5

Dust, Mites, Moulds, Animals and Pollens

Know Thine Enemy

There is a universal agreement that these biological inhaled particles are the most common cause of asthma. As they are, therefore, for many asthma sufferers the 'enemy', it is important to identify them for the individual sufferer and help him or her to make plans to defeat that enemy. Often modification to the home environment can lead to an enormous improvement in asthma and enable a major reduction in the usage of medication.

Many asthmatics know, without any recourse to skin testing, that their asthma is enormously influenced by contact with dust, dust mites, moulds, animals, feathers and pollens. They observe that they wheeze when dusting a room, when turning over a compost heap, when raking leaves, when sleeping on a feather pillow and when in close contact with animals such as cats and dogs. Others notice that their asthma only occurs in the grass or tree pollen seasons of the year. They may also observe that when they go abroad to a hot, dry climate such as is found in the Greek islands, the Balearic islands, the Portugese Algarve, etc., their asthma disappears. In these localities the contact with dust, dust mites and moulds is vastly decreased.

In some asthmatics, though, the cause-and-effect relationship with aero-allergens is not that obvious. Some will not react at all to these items, but will react to various foods they are consuming. In these circumstances skin testing is vital in identifying the problem. For some patients ordinary prick testing is a reasonably satisfactory procedure, but it gives negative responses at times even when it is known for certain that the sufferer is definitely reacting to a specific aero-allergen. Drops of housedust mite, for example, may be instilled into the nasal passages and produce an asthmatic result, yet a skin test will still register 'negative'.

Any physician using intradermal provocation skin testing knows why this should be: the short answer is that the prick test solutions are too weak. With prick testing a large number of allergens are all tested at the same time, and if the extracts used were stronger the patient could well have a severe reaction to the procedure.

In contrast, with intradermal provocation testing a single allergen like dust mite is injected and the injection given intradermally (that is, between the layers of skin) as opposed to being pricked into the skin. Intradermal test solutions are produced in various concentrations, with a dilution factor of 5 between each concentration. The 1-in-5 dilution of the concentrated extract is called the 'Number 1' level. The 1-in-25 dilution is called the 'Number 2' level, the 1-in-125 dilution is the 'Number 3' level and the 1-in-625 dilution is called the 'Number 4' level. Frequently, dilutions such as '5', '6', '7', '8' and '9' are also employed.

Clinical observations show that giving the 'Number 4' level (1-in-625 strength) is equivalent to a skin prick test. Thus if such a test is positive the 'Number 4' level intradermal will also be positive. What is seen daily when intradermal provocation testing is employed, is patients showing negative on the 'Number 4' level but positive on either the 'Number 2' or 'Number 3' levels. Frequently a patient will show a positive wheal, for example, on the 'Number 2' level, associated quite often with symptoms of asthma, while the 'Number 3' or 'Number 4' level may be negative. The strongest negative wheal is called the *neutralizing dose*; when this dose is given the symptoms abate. This is the foundation of neutralization treatment and will be explained in much greater depth in Chapters 12 and 13.

Dust and Dust Mite

The most common and important inhaled allergen, which can affect people throughout the year, is the housedust mite. In the UK the most common type is called *Dermatophagoides pyteronnisius*. The term 'dermatophagoides' means skin-eater: this microscopic organism feeds off discarded human skin flakes which we are shedding every moment of our lives. These skin particles consist of a protein called keratin, which itself is colonized by moulds, yeasts and bacteria. Thus, the dust mite is largely dependent on us human beings for their very existence. There are more than 2 million housedust mites found in the average double mattress, and it has been calculated that 10 per cent of the weight of an average pillow consists of dead skin and housedust mites. As these dust mites defecate about 20 times a day, this is not a particularly appetizing thought. Interestingly, it has been estimated that if all the housedust mites in an average double bed were laid out nose to tail, they would stretch the length of five football stadiums. Of course, bedding mattresses and pillows are the soft furnishings with which we human beings have the most constant and intimate contact. We spend an average of about eight hours a day in bed, and while in bed we are warm and frequently sweating. Dust mites take about four weeks to develop from eggs into adults, and live for up to 40 days. The inhaled particles that cause asthma are not the mite itself but its faecal droppings. These are very small and light and easily become airborne and remain airborne for a long time. Humidity is absolutely vital for the health and survival of dust mites, and so the pillow moistened by our damp breath throughout the night is the ideal place for these creatures to flourish. Above the pillow there is a cloud of minute faecal particles queueing up to enter our nasal passages and lungs. No wonder so many asthmatics have such wheezy nights.

The vast increase in hermetic heat insulation in modern houses could not suit the dust mite more. In old, draughty houses it has a much greater problem with survival, so ventilating the house at frequent intervals is a helpful move in containing the levels of these organisms.

Houses with above-average moisture, like those near rivers, lakes and the sea, will probably have a higher dust mite content than others. Of course, these same circumstances will also encourage moulds, and may confuse the diagnosis slightly.

A profusion of other soft furnishings, such as wall-to-wall carpeting, sofas, armchairs and so on, can contribute to the dust mite problem. Apart from reacting to the dust mite droppings, many people react to other components of housedust. Allergists normally skin test separately for housedust and housedust mite. Household dust is a complex mixture of many things, containing such items as moulds, mould spores, fragments of insects such as house flies, carpet beetles, and cockroach particles. These have been identified in some housedust samples even when there was no evidence of cockroach infestation in the house.

Dealing with Dust and Dust Mite Sensitivity

In many patients the single most effective technique is neutralization therapy, because although we can make many suggestions about reducing contact with these organisms in the house, it is still going to be contacted at the workplace, schools, the cinema and in other people's homes. Modification of the domestic environment, however, may be especially effective with a young child, who may spend 90 per cent of the time within the home. Adults can also notice a big improvement, as the worse contact they have throughout any 24 hours is through their bedding mattress and pillows.

There are a whole range of 'weapons' which can be used in the battle against the housedust mite. The most effective are:

• mattress and pillow enclosures
• acaricide sprays and liquid nitrogen
• special vacuum cleaners
• damp-dusting and airing of bedrooms
• air filters.

The most important single move that can be made against the housedust mite is to enclose your mattress and pillows in microporous covers. These let water vapour through but act as a very effective barrier to dust mites and their droppings. The older, plastic mattress covers were completely impermeable and a drop in temperature would produce condensation on the inside of these covers. This in turn could lead to the growth of moulds, which would become a big problem if any holes appeared in the cover. Furthermore, microporous covers are not slippery the way plastic ones are, so bedding sheets remain where they are supposed to be. These covers are also available for duvets and the box springs in the base of the bed.

The Intervent range of microporous mattress covers manufactured by Slumberland can be obtained from certain specialist pharmacies. Specialist suppliers of these products include Allerayde and The Healthy House (*see Useful Addresses*). The cost of these mattress enclosures are not cheap but do vary quite quite a lot. A pillowcase can, for example, cost anywhere between £8 ($12) and £25 ($37). A double duvet cover can cost between £25 ($37) and £150 ($225) and a double mattress cover between £36 ($48) and £140 ($210), at the time of writing.

Acaracides and Liquid Nitrogen

With these covers in place it doesn't matter whether the mattress itself is of traditional interior spring design or of foam rubber. Similarly, the covers do not need to be vacuumed frequently. It is ideal to fit the covers onto a brand new mattress – some suppliers sell new mattresses which are sealed in with microporous covering during the manufacturing process. If buying a new mattress is out of the question, there are ways of reducing the mites in an existing mattress prior to sealing it with a microporous cover. One is to use an acaricide spray, which kills both dust mites and ticks. Dust mites are related to spiders (arachnoids). In common with spiders, dust mites have eight legs. Dust mites and ticks are in the same zoological order, called acari. Thus the chemicals that kill both ticks and dust mites are termed acaricides. (For information on suppliers of acaricides including Crawford Pharmaceuticals and C.D. Searle *see Useful Addresses*.) Crawford Pharmaceuticals sell the Acarosan range, the active ingredient of which is benzyl benzoate. Foam in spray cans is supplied for mattresses and upholstery, whereas a moist powder is used for carpets. Searle Consumer Products produce and sell the Actomite range. The active ingredients are two synthetic pyrethroids.

For either of these products the amount needed to treat an average living room and bedroom would cost around £40 ($60) and this treatment would be needed twice a year.

With any acaricide it is essential that the treatment is followed by a really thorough vacuum cleaning. Not only does one need to kill the dust mites, but also to remove their corpses and all their old faecal droppings.

A very effective acaricide treatment is liquid nitrogen. Liquid nitrogen is extremely cold and freezes the mites to death. Currently, to my knowledge, there are no nationwide suppliers of this treatment in the UK, although there is a firm called C.B.C. (*see Useful Addresses*) who can help people in London and the Home Counties, but not elsewhere. Therefore the provision of this service is somewhat patchy throughout the United Kingdom. Treatment is fairly inexpensive. Usually they also treat the carpet immediately adjacent to the bed. Liquid nitrogen does not damage carpets or upholstery, but as it is extremely cold it has to be handled by trained personnel. This treatment needs to be repeated approximately every six months and the contractors can give the rooms a good vacuuming after they have completed the initial treatment. Dust mites, however, gradually find their way back into the house via the clothes people wear, and so the treatment needs to be repeated.

Some may wonder whether just enclosing the mattress and pillows may be sufficient, and indeed it is for some patients. If, however, the dust mites are enclosed by the microporous covers, they will be locked in with their food supply and continue to breed. If any minute holes develop in the covers, they will seep out and possibly cause problems at a later date.

Vacuum Cleaners

Most ordinary vacuum cleaners are pretty useless at reducing dust mite exposure. The collecting bags have small pores which allow the dust mite droppings to escape. They then leave the vacuum cleaner via the exhaust, often increasing the amount of allergen in the air.

Special vacuum cleaners designed specifically for this problem are now available. They use better bags, which retain the allergic particles, and are backed up by a high-quality filter that cleans the exhaust gas before it leaves the machine. They also have much more powerful suction power than other cleaners.

A cheaper alternative is to fit a pad of filter material to your existing vacuum cleaner, though this will not give such good results.

Allerayde, mentioned earlier, sell the NILFISK vacuum cleaner and VACUFILT exhaust filters for conventional vacuum cleaners.

Medivac sell a vacuum cleaner that contains a Hepa filter. It retains 99.97 per cent of particles at 0.3 microns. Recently, Medivac have added the 'Medivap Home Asthma Treatment' to their range. This is a treatment which uses electronically pressurized steam to be forced deep into carpets, mattresses and upholstery, destroying dust mites, cat fleas, bacteria and other living organisms. Furthermore, it has been shown in clinical trials that it combines the destruction of mites and also their faecal droppings, which are the major asthma trigger. Dr. Matthew Colloff of the University of Glasgow, one of the world's leading authorities on dust mites, has stated that this is the only method of housedust mite control that combines effective killing of mites and a substantial reduction in allergen concentration within a single system.

Nilfisk Limited sell the Allergy Vac vacuum cleaner, which contains a Hepa filter. It retains 99.97 per cent of particles at 0.3 microns.

All of these makes have been independently tested with good results. These vacuum cleaner prices start at around £300 ($450) and in addition to that one will need replacement filters from time to time on some machines.

Allerayde, The Healthy House and Medivac (*see Useful Addresses*) all stock a wide range of dust mite enclosure materials, vacuum cleaners, acaricide sprays, etc.

Dehumidifiers

These machines are useful for reducing the humidity which is so vital to the survival of dust mites. For convenience they are discussed in detail in the section on moulds (*see page 45*).

Damp-dusting

Damp-dusting with a wet cloth, as opposed to flitting around the room with a feather duster, is a simple yet effective way of reducing dust levels in the home.

Air Filters

There are three types of machines used to clean air: ionizers, electro-static air cleaners, and Hepa filter air cleaners.

Ionizers are inexpensive but are generally too small to make any noticeable improvement in air quality. There has been no convincing medical evidence to show that ionizers improve air quality in people suffering from asthma. In fact, the ionization process can produce ozone, which can then trigger an asthma attack.

Electrostatic air cleaners effectively remove smoke and they are thus popular in pubs and restaurants. However, they require regular cleaning and have a very limited effect on bacteria, viruses and odours. Their test efficiency is only estimated at 70 per cent.

Hepa filter air cleaners force the air through a filter which physically traps airborne pollutants. The greater the surface area of the Hepa filter, the better it performs. The best quality Hepa filters bring the greatest benefit to asthma and allergy sufferers; some meet with 99.97 per cent efficiency in terms of removing the 0.3 micron particle.

Honeywell Envirocare Air Filters are amongst the best models available. Their phone number is given in the Useful Addresses chapter.

The air filters I have personally been acquainted with seem rather noisy to me and I would find it difficult to sleep with the noise of one in my bedroom. These filters are, I think, worth a try for a few weeks on approval, if other steps have failed to deliver the required results.

Thus, to summarize the environmental control of dust and dust mite, we could say that:

1. The quickest, cheapest and most effective measure is the use of microporous covers for the bed.
2. Regular airing of the bed and the bedroom, combined with wet dusting, are both cheap and very effective.
3. A specialized vacuum cleaner is very helpful.
4. The various forms of acaricide treatment are well worth considering.

How aggressively one goes about this depends entirely on how sensitive the individual sufferer is to the problem. I should emphasize that these techniques are of no value unless housedust and dust mite are the main culprits in bringing on your asthma symptoms.

Moulds

Many people have very little knowledge or appreciation of the existence of moulds in the air that we breathe. In fact, there are more mould spores in the air than any other component. Numerically, there are about 50 times more mould spores in the atmosphere than there is grass pollen during the pollen season. The most obvious evidence of the existence of moulds is the green discolouration on stale bread and the furry covering on old fruit and vegetables. In the countryside they cover all rotting leaves, fruit and the wood of dead trees. Apart from feeding on all this organic matter, moulds are able to feed on other particular matter floating in the atmosphere.

In damp houses problems with moulds can exist all year round, especially with the mould penicillum, which is the one responsible for the green appearance on stale bread.

Outdoor moulds have a distinct season during which they can cause problems. Moulds needs warmth and humidity to survive, and are most prevalent from midsummer to early Autumn. One of the four most prevalent moulds in the UK is *Cladosporium herbarum*, which begins its spore production in June. This leads to possible diagnostic confusion with grass pollens, which have the same season of pollination.

In the UK there are about 20 different moulds which can cause mischief; most allergy clinics have facilities to test them all. The major outdoor moulds that we test for routinely are *Alternaria alternata*, *Cephalosporium*, *Aspergillae* and *Cladosporium*. These specific moulds have been selected on the basis of their prevalence and capacity to cause trouble. Apart from skin testing, mould sensitivity can be suspected and frequently diagnosed by the patient's observations of when symptoms are worse or better. Typically, a mould-sensitive patient may notice that wheezing is particularly bad when:

- compost heaps are turned over: when this happens a huge cloud of mould spores is emitted
- leaves are raked
- it is warm, humid or rainy, and especially when the sufferer is near deciduous trees
- just before a thunderstorm, as the massive rises in humidity induces sporelation of moulds
- near to harvesting: especially a combine harvester. These machines create a massive cloud of mould spores in their wake.

Conversely, a mould-sensitive patient will be *much improved*:

- on hot, very dry days in summer, and especially while on holiday in hot, dry climes like the Greek islands or any desert environment
- after the first major frost of the winter, which after a few days reduces the mould count enormously
- on a winter holiday in the mountains.

People who have problems with the housedust mite are also improved markedly if holidays are taken more than 600 miles south of London. At latitudes nearing the equator there are no dust mites. Moulds are much more difficult to avoid than dust and dust mites, because it is impossible to control outdoor pollution other than by emigration; desensitization by the neutralization technique really is the most important part of combating this particular problem. However, things can be done to reduce indoor mould pollution.

Dealing with Indoor Mould Pollution

To reduce this pollution steps may be taken:

1. to minimize the amount of dampness that gets into the house
2. to reduce moisture production within the house, and condensation
3. to eliminate other sources of mould and to kill existing moulds.

Minimizing the Amount of Dampness that Enters the House

Many householders are familiar with the sudden appearance of a damp patch on the inside of exterior walls. This is usually due to rain water penetrating the mortar or bricks and permeating through to the inside of the wall. Obviously the advice of a competent builder or surveyor should be sought in these circumstances, but often a coating of silicone can be sprayed on the outside wall. This is invisible and usually highly effective.

Rising damp is common in very old houses, especially those built before 1920. Many of these houses have no damp course which acts as a barrier to rising damp. This can be corrected by injecting a silicone compound into a row of small holes just above ground level. This silicone hardens and forms a waterproof layer. These chemical damp courses are very effective and usually solve the problem.

If any damp spot is exposed to dry heat and light, both disapproved of by moulds, there is usually a prompt resolution of the problem.

One of the more expensive problems is the discovery that water is seeping up from the ground through the floors. This may require a whole new floor and the incorporation of a layer of waterproof material before it is laid.

Reducing Moisture Production and Condensation within the House

Moisture is produced in large amounts within the house from human beings themselves, from steaming kettles, boiling vegetables, drying clothes, showers and baths. Steps that can be taken to help include:

- covering pots of boiling vegetables or other foods
- drying clothes out of doors whenever possible, or using a tumble dryer
- taking baths rather than showers
- airing the house as frequently as possible to allow moisture to escape, especially when the outside air is dry
- mopping up any condensation that occurs on window sills, and removing any signs of mould growth
- possibly using an extractor fan in the kitchen or bathroom, as condensation is pretty well unavoidable in these rooms
- using dehumidifiers
- using air conditioners.

People with mould or dust mite sensitivity should never use a humidifier. Increased humidity is the worst possible scenario. Reduced humidity is what is required, and dehumidifiers can be very effective in this respect.

All humidifiers use the same technology as refrigerators and work by cooling air. As air cools, water condenses out of it and is collected in a tank within the dehumidifier, from which the water is unable to evaporate. Dry, cool air then leaves the machine and is heated up again by contact with the warm air in the room. Usually the water tank needs to be removed and emptied about once a day.

For more information, contact Beta Plus, the Healthy House or Medivac (*see Useful Addresses*).

Relatively low-powered dehumidifiers are sold widely in stores such as Curry's, but specialist firms sell more powerful models.

Beta Plus sell a good range of dehumidifiers that reduce relative humidity to 45 per cent. They also sell an expensive meter which can measure humidity in domestic circumstances.

Medivac sell what is possibly the 'Rolls Royce' of dehumidifiers, which is called the Banamite Enviro Dry Dehumidifier. This also incorporates an electrostatic microfilter which helps to remove mite droppings, mould spores and pollen from the air. This particular dehumidifier costs around £400 ($600), but some of the other alternatives are available for between £200 ($350) and £300 ($450).

Air Conditioners will achieve a lot of what dehumidifiers can, though they are considerably more expensive and, depending on where you live, may not be the most cost-effective solution.

Eliminating Other Sources of Mould and Killing Existing Moulds
Sensible and easy precautions:

- Make sure that no food is allowed to go mouldy within the house. Anything that does should be thrown out immediately.
- Pot plants are a potent source of mould growth, especially those that need to be kept damp all the time. Artificial plants or cactii are a much better bet.
- Wash shower curtains frequently.
- Clean the rubber seals around fridges and freezers. Lots of mould finds its way into the crevices in these seals.
- Use a mould-retardent solution for the bottoms of windows, bathroom tiles, vinyl baths, etc. (Allerayde is one supplier: *see Useful Addresses.*)

Allerayde sell mildew remover at approximately £8 ($12) a bottle. They also sell the Mildew Stop aerosol (£7/$10.50 a bottle) which is effective in preventing mould regrowth on carpets and curtains.

Animals

Cats

Cats are by far the biggest offenders for asthmatic patients. However, many other asthmatics have problems with dogs, horses, hamsters, gerbils, guinea pigs, rats and mice (goldfish are quite safe!). Most people who have a problem with cats are very well aware of it; for some, even the smallest amount of allergen carried on the clothes of a pet owner is enough to set off an attack.

When a cat licks itself the air is filled with microscopic specks of dried saliva which contain a protein that is the main allergen for those affected by cats. This protein spreads itself everywhere, coating the walls, windows and furniture. As the particles are very small and light they stay airborne for many hours. Cat salivary protein can be detected even when a cat has vacated a house for several years, and so if the decision is made, somewhat reluctantly, to ask your furry friend politely to depart, a thorough cleaning of the house is still needed. This means washing all the curtains and fabrics, having the carpets shampooed and the walls washed.

Desensitization by the neutralization technique can enable a number of patients, particularly with milder asthma, to retain their cats, but if cat contact is leading to severe asthmatic reactions it is quite definitely better to part company. Other procedures that can help with milder cases are:

- excluding the cat from the bedroom of the asthmatic sufferer
- frequent ventilation of the house
- suggesting to the cat that he or she spend more time outdoors
- washing and shampooing the cat thoroughly once a week (this substantially reduces the amount of allergen available)
- washing the cat's blanket weekly (a well lived-in cat's blanket can contain the most astronomic amount of allergen!)

Dogs

In general, these are less of a problem than cats, but they still constitute a very major dilemma for some people. The allergens are present in skin particles and in the saliva. These allergenic particles become attached to the fur, which is not allergenic in itself. If the problem is bad enough, the dog may reluctantly have to go, though this will undoubtedly be a very emotionally difficult decision. Many dog-owners will prefer to get by with a combination of neutralization and measures similar to those mentioned above for cats.

Summer Pollens

When summer pollens are a part or the whole of the problem, it is usually fairly obvious to both the asthma sufferer and his or her physician. Asthma related solely to pollen sensitivity is restricted entirely to the 'season' of that pollen. A diagnosis of which specific pollen is involved can usually be made by carefully chronicling the months in which asthma occurs. This is reasonably easy when the asthma is entirely related to the summer months, but much more hazardous when all-year-round allergens are operating at the same time.

As a general rule, if a patient has symptoms limited to the spring, the culprits are usually tree pollens. The most common trees involved are Beech, Birch, Alder, Oak, Hazel, Ash, Plane and Poplar trees. These trees are all 'wind pollenated' and the pollen is very widely distributed by the wind. It is said that some tree pollens can travel up to 100 miles on the wind. In contrast, trees that have exotic blooms are 'insect pollenated': their beautiful floral appearance attracts insects which then effectively transfer the pollens themselves. Cherry trees are a good example of an insect pollenated tree; its pollen rarely gives human beings any problems unless they are literally standing under the tree. Most allergy clinics carry individual extracts of the major wind pollenating trees, so the individual's specific sensitivities can be pinpointed.

Identification of specific grass, tree, weed or shrub involvement is only really important if the neutralization form of desensitization is going to be employed. If the only treatment contemplated is drug treatment by mast cell stabilizers, antihistamines, steroids or beta-2 antagonists, then the source of the problem is pretty well irrelevant. As these are the usual approaches to the treatment of asthma caused by summer pollens it explains why most physicians are not interested in the source of the problem. Whereas in hayfever, anti-histamines are the main stay of treatment, in asthma anti-histamines are not particularly helpful, as asthma is a more complex reaction involving mediators other than histamine.

Asthma which occurs predominantly in early to mid-summer is nearly always caused by grass pollens, though some early sporing moulds can cause confusion in this respect. A very small number of sufferers have problems late in summer, which are usually caused by reactions to nettles, mugwort, plantains or dock pollen.

Ordinary standard skin prick tests are fairly reliable in diagnosing allergies to summer pollens, as opposed to mould reactions and food sensitivity. When a prick test is used to identify a summer pollen, a small amount of the specific pollen is injected into the skin to observe what reaction occurs. A positive reaction shows that the allergy antibody, IgE, is present in the skin and that particular IgE is specific for that pollen. It doesn't conclusively show that the patient has hayfever as a result of that specific pollen. However, if there is IgE present to that pollen in the skin it is very probable that identical IgE antibodies exist within the nose, though this is not 100 per cent certain.

Thus, skin tests are not the 'be all and end all' of allergy diagnosis; for an accurate diagnosis they have to be considered in concert with evidence of the timing of the asthmatic symptoms. As in diagnosing the all-year-round allergies, the intradermal provocative test, although more time-consuming, does in fact have a higher degree of accuracy.

Figure 9 offers a general guide to the main pollen seasons of the various trees, grasses, weeds and shrubs in the United Kingdom. These pollens can exist in extremely low concentrations just outside the seasons indicated.

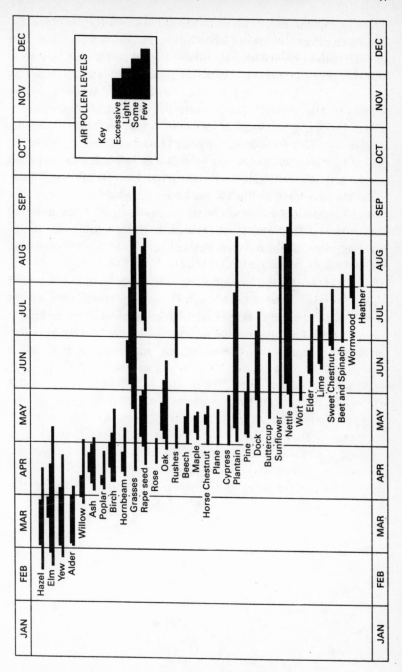

Figure 9 Pollen calendar

The potential for structural changes in the home or the use of specialized machines is very limited when one is dealing with problems with summer pollens. Most patients who suffer from these allergies know full well that they can wake up early on a summer day and be streaming or wheezing, despite tightly closed windows. Air-conditioning systems certainly do remove a substantial amount of these summer pollens. Adding a high-quality air filtration unit to the intake on air-conditioning systems reduces the pollen count to about 2 per cent of the outdoor level. Of course, even if this does help it leaves the pollen sufferer fearful of venturing forth into the outside world. A long holiday in the Mediterranean may be a better bet on the whole.

Air filters and ionizers almost certainly remove significant amounts of pollen from the air, and some sufferers have reported good results. However, many do not and there has been very little scientific validation of their benefit.

Neutralization/desensitization is the only technique that I have seen produce very good results. Although I am not personally acquainted with it, some physicians have reported good results using a technique called Enzyme Potentiated Desensitization. My own severe tree pollen sensitivity responded excellently (thank goodness) to tree pollen neutralization.

Food Sensitivity and Asthma

First, there are two myths commonly held by patients (and many physicians) that need dispelling concerning food sensitivity.

Myth 1: The problem cannot be food, as I hadn't changed my diet when the asthma started.
Myth 2: If I had a food sensitivity, I would surely have observed it.

Regarding *Myth 1*, only about 3 per cent of all food sensitivities exist in sufferers from birth. These are termed *fixed food sensitivities* and the reaction is usually to rarely consumed and exotic foods. These reactions are the ones that everyone is aware of. The other 97 per cent of food sensitivities develop insidiously with the passage of time, and are usually to foods consumed very frequently, such as wheat, corn, rye, oats, milk, beef, beet sugar, cane sugar, eggs, soy, coffee, tea and yeast.

The most well-known allergy of all is of course hayfever, and the vast majority of people who suffer from this condition start in their late teens or early twenties. These people have inhaled grass pollens for many years before they start to react to them. Similarly, middle-aged, late onset asthma patients have inhaled dust, dust mite and moulds for maybe over 40 years before developing a problem with them.

Going on to *Myth 2*, virtually no one who has food sensitivity knows it. The foods involved are, as I have just said, everyday ones, and the phenomenon of masking, described in depth later in Chapter 6, ensures that we do not spot them. Masking refers to the phenomenon in which repeated doses of an allergic food first make a patient feel better before he or she feels worse. A further dose then improves the patient again, just like a further dose of scotch whisky will initially make the alcoholic feel better.

There is much dispute amongst physicians of different persuasions as to whether we should at this point be talking about sensitivity, intolerance or allergy. There will be a discussion of the merits of these various terms later on in this chapter.

Any physician who has tried putting a wide range of patients through well-designed elimination diets knows that food sensitivity is a very major cause of asthma. In fact, after reactions to airborne allergens such as dust, dust mite, moulds and animal danders, it is the next most common cause of asthma.

Historically, asthma has been divided by chest physicians into *extrinsic asthma* and *intrinsic asthma*.

Extrinsic asthma is diagnosed when the patient gives a clear history of reactions to airborne allergens, usually accompanied by positive skin prick tests to those allergens. Those who do not are usually labelled as having intrinsic asthma, which really means nothing unless one includes unexplainable acts of God.

The vast majority of patients who are diagnosed as suffering from intrinsic asthma are in fact suffering from food sensitivity. The main reason why food sensitivity has not been diagnosed frequently in the past is that such sensitivity is not commonly diagnosable by conventional skin prick tests. In fact, skin prick tests have been shown to be positive in only 15 per cent of known food sensitivities. Thus, this test is 85 per cent unreliable, which makes it a definite source of misinformation. To emphasize this unreliability, one can say that tossing a coin is over three times more reliable than skin prick testing, as this does at least lead to a 50 per cent success rate.

In contrast, intradermal provocative neutralization testing, described in Chapters 12, 13 and 14, has a high reliability rate.

Elimination diets are the best method by which doctors and patients can observe the relationship between food and their asthma. Unfortunately, very few physicians have attempted to observe these phenomena and prefer to content themselves with skin prick tests, RAST tests or cytotoxic tests, all of which have very major degrees of unreliability. What is much more reliable is to put the patient on a collection of about 10 to 15 foods that have a very good track record when it comes to food sensitivity, and keep them on this diet for seven days. The change that can occur in a patient with food sensitivity while on such a diet is one of the most satisfying things that a physician can witness. Patients are astonished that within a few days of being on such a diet they can omit their inhalers and other symptom-suppressive drugs. After observing this dramatic improvement the patient can reintroduce foods one at a time back into his or her diet and observe which foods produce no problem and which foods produce an asthmatic reaction. Some people object to this procedure because it is fairly slow and takes several weeks, and is rather anti-social for the first two or three weeks. However, when one realizes that one is trying to resolve a problem which may be life-long, this is a very small price to pay. Many patients cease to have asthma at all after such a procedure and can forget their daily doses of a wide variety of drugs. It is far, far better to discover the causes of problems than continually to suppress them by various drug treatments. The details of the Asthma Elimination Diet are in Chapter 11; in that chapter I will go into the practical details of how to sort out food sensitivity. The rest of this chapter is concerned with the rules of food sensitivity and the various theoretical concepts about the way it works.

The physician who has done more than anyone else, in my opinion, to document the inter-relationship between food sensitivity and asthma is Dr. Derek Wraith, who until he retired was Consultant Physician to the Chest Department at St. Thomas' Hospital in London.

Dr. Derek Wraith has published his research into 265 patients with asthma found to be caused by foods or food additives. Just over half of these patients were under 15 years old. There were more males (65 per cent) in the younger group and, interestingly, far more females (75 per cent) in the over-15 group.

The asthma in these patients was quite severe: 26 per cent of them were on continuous or intermittent steroids, and 44 per cent were on regular bronchodilators. After avoiding incriminated foods, the number using steroids dropped to 3 per cent, and the number using regular bronchodilators dropped to 20 per cent.

I might at this point mention that many patients whose asthma is due partly to food sensitivity also have inhalant sensitivities, for example to dust, dust mites and moulds, and I imagine that a fair number of these patients had a bit of both. Dr. Wraith didn't have access to neutralization treatment for airborne allergens, but one can see that with just the food allergy management there was a considerable decrease in the expense and inconvenience of drug treatment.

Figure 10 shows the main foods found to cause asthma in those younger than 15 and aged 15 and above.

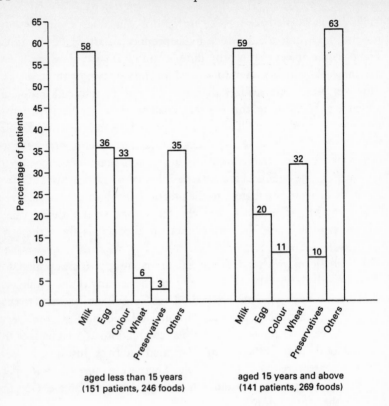

Figure 10

In the younger age group, milk, eggs and artificial colourants stood out as being the chief culprits, whereas in the older group there was a much wider range of incriminated foods. Milk was still the most common single culprit, but wheat made a major contribution as well. However, it must be emphasized that in both age groups virtually any food could be a problem. Dr. Wraith emphasizes, quite rightly, that in those adults who were sensitive to wheat, other cereals, especially corn, rye and oats, were also frequently implicated.

Artificial colourants played a large role in the younger patients, as young children tend to eat a lot of foods highly contaminated by such chemicals, such as soft drinks, sweets, ice creams, cakes and so forth. These artificial colourants are also widely used in medications.

I have selected two cases (Figures 11 and 12) from Dr. Wraith's studies which will give a general flavour of the findings he reported.[1] The peak flow readings mentioned in these studies will be familiar to most patients with asthma, many of whom will have blown into these devices on many occasions. Peak flow meters simply measure the speed at which breath can be exhaled from the lungs. If there is substantial spasm in the bronchial tubes, this rate is markedly decreased.

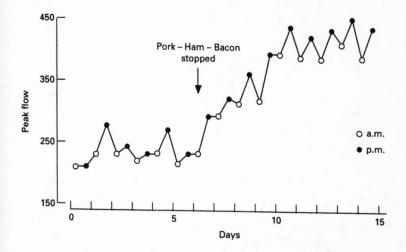

Figure 11 Male, 40 years: morning and evening peak flow breathing tests and a diary of all foods, etc. The patient showed improved values when pork, ham and bacon were stopped. Several other allergenic foods were found later and all were confirmed by a fall in peak flow values on their reintroduction. From Wraith, with permission.

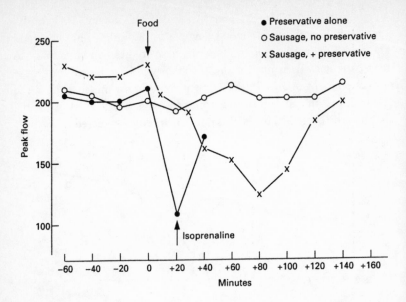

Figure 12 Female, 57 years, with recent onset of severe asthma considered to be 'intrinsic'. Skin tests were negative. Food tests confirmed preservatives as the cause. There was a rapid and big drop in peak flow values and severe breathlessness after lemonade containing preservatives (sodium benzoate and sulphur dioxide). On other days, sausages with identical appearances with and without preservatives caused fall (O)and no fall (x) in peak flow values. From Wraith, with permission.

As can be seen in Figure 12, when the preservative was given by itself the reduction in peak flow was so extreme that Isoprenaline had to be administered to 'rescue' the patient.

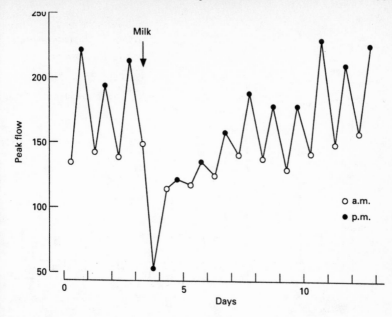

Figure 13 Male, 55 years, with 15 years, persistent and severe asthma causing much disability and necessitating steroid therapy. Skin tests for inhalants and foods were negative. Symptoms improved on stopping milk and deteriorated on restarting it. The figure shows a fall in peak flow values which persisted for a week after taking half a pint of milk only. From Wraith, with permission.

Dr. Wraith has made hundreds of similar observations on his patients. These findings cannot just be ignored.

Amongst other reports illustrating the importance of food allergy and intolerance in asthma are those of Rowe,[2] Gerrard,[3] Oggle & Bullock,[4] Papageorgiou et al.,[5] Kniker & Rodriguez,[6] Dahl & Zeteerstrom,[7] and Dahl.[8] Additives in foods, artificial colourings and preservatives have been shown to be causes of asthma by Stenius & Lemola,[9] Freedman,[10,11] Baker et al.,[12] Stevenson and Simon,[13] and Ortolani et al.[14]

Aside from asthma, the majority (65 per cent) of patients in Dr. Wraith's study had other symptoms, often several caused by foods (*see Figure 14*).

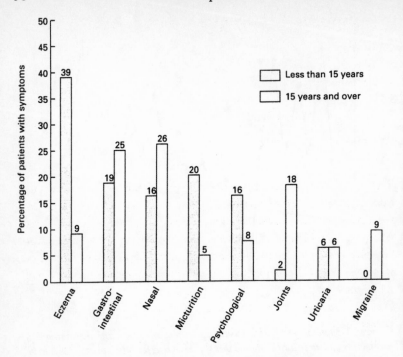

Figure 14 Other symptoms. The figure shows the percentages of the different symptoms in the younger and older age groups. Under 15 years 102 patients (67%) and over 15 years, 114 patients (64%) had one or more symptoms.

The fact that the food-sensitive patient often has several different problems is emphasized because their combination is a characteristic feature of food sensitivity and hence has some diagnostic value. These observations emphasize what a huge role food allergy, sensitivity or intolerance play in human illness.

When Dr. Wraith did these studies he was well aware of the most important fact about food sensitivity, which is the concept of *masking*. Masking means that when a food such as wheat or milk is eaten regularly it will give, on ingestion, no obvious adverse reaction. In fact, each ingestion causes possibly a slight improvement in the symptoms, and as a result the patient is totally unaware of the role that that food is playing in his or her problem. A helpful analogy is with the alcoholic, whose ingestion of alcohol may well be the cause of his or her long-term problems, but in the short term another 'dose' seems to make him feel much better.

Important Concepts in Food Sensitivity

1. Masking
2. Adaptation
3. Fixed and Cyclic Food Sensitivities
4. Defining Allergy
5. The Rotary Diversified Diet

Masking

There is no more important concept to grasp about food sensitivity than masking, because this explains why almost everyone who has a food sensitivity problem is totally unaware of it. Such people assume, totally wrongly, that if they did have a food sensitivity it would become completely obvious to them. Most people are familiar with and understand the idea that someone can be sensitive to a food eaten occasionally. The public concept of food allergy has mostly been related to foods that are exotic or eaten only occasionally. Unhappily, many physicians still take this exceedingly simplistic view of food sensitivity.

The concept of masked food allergy was originally identified by Dr. Herbert Rinkel, a well-known allergist practising in Oklahoma City. Dr. Rinkel was renowned for being an extremely acute observer of various cause-and-effect relationships. After he qualified in medicine he developed a severe nasal allergy called allergic rhinitis, which is a condition characterized by severe, persistent nasal discharge. His medical colleagues skin-tested him for all the well-known inhalant allergies and these tests proved negative.

Dr. Rinkel was familiar with Dr. Rowe's work on food allergy and suspected he might have such a problem himself. When he had been a medical student, like many of his colleagues he had been fairly impecunious. Rinkel's father, who was an egg farmer, had tried to help his son out during his medical studentship by sending him a gross of eggs (144) each week; this was the main source of protein for young Rinkel and his family. This high ingestion of eggs continued after he qualified, and he therefore suspected eggs as a cause of his problem. One afternoon, in an attempt to produce an adverse reaction he consumed a large quantity of eggs, but to his surprise his nasal symptoms on that afternoon were, if anything rather improved. Some years later he did the opposite – he abstained from eggs for about five days, and then discovered that his nasal discharge improved very considerably. After five days he inadvertently consumed some egg (in an angel cake) at a birthday party. He suddenly collapsed unconscious and his rhinitis returned in dramatic fashion.

Dr. Rinkel conceived as a result of this experience that he might well have stumbled on something fundamental regarding the basic nature of food allergy. He thus repeated the experiment by re-establishing his consumption of eggs, omitting them again for five days and again repeating the egg ingestion, which caused a recurrence of the symptoms of unconsciousness and nasal discharge. He next extended his observations to a number of his patients, and found a similar phenomenon occurring with a wide variety of different foods and with a wide variety of medical conditions, including asthma. His observations were first published in 1944, where masking was defined in the following way:

> If a person ingests a particular food each day he or she may become allergic to it and yet not suspect this as a cause of the symptoms. It is usual to feel better after a meal than before. In this case, the feedings tend to mask the symptoms of the allergic response.

Dr. Rinkel could not explain his observations.

Since Dr. Rinkel's original work, cases of masked food allergy have been reported in many thousands of patients. Masked food allergy represents an interesting model of addictive behaviour and is, in my opinion, the major basic mechanism behind the addiction to such apparently diverse items as coffee, tea, sugar, alcoholic beverages, and tobacco. This concept can be represented graphically, as shown in Figure 15.

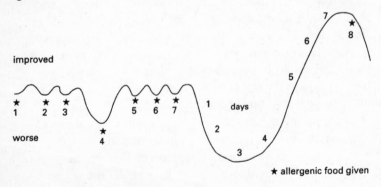

Figure 15 Masked Food Allergy

Figure 15 illustrates the results of eating or not eating a masked food allergen in someone with a single food allergy. Each asterisk represents the feeding of the allergenic food. As can be seen, the second feeding aborts the deterioration of symptoms which is seen after the first feeding. This is followed by an improvement. A similar response is experienced after the third feeding. Because the fourth feeding of the allergenic food is delayed, the response is further down the withdrawal curve and is thus worse. Following this fourth feeding, the person's condition usually returns to normal.

After the seventh feeding, in this example, the subject has been told to avoid the allergenic food and then exhibits the classic withdrawal phenomenon, characterized by a considerable worsening of symptoms, usually by the evening of the first day. These symptoms may be of headache, fatigue or joint pain. The second and third days tend to be quite severe, but they are followed by a slow improvement until the sixth day. By the sixth day most people are symptom-free if under 35 years old. In those who are older than 35, the symptoms may take another day or so to clear. It is extremely gratifying to see someone with constant asthma clear of symptoms for the first time for several years on the sixth or seventh day of this withdrawal period. Feeding after the seventh day (*8 in Figure 15) represents a deliberate re-feeding of the avoided food and the Rinkel hyperacute response. In this, as illustrated by Rinkel's experience, symptoms return quickly and quite dramatically.

Figure 15 demonstrates how complicated is the relationship between one commonly-eaten food allergen and the symptomatology that it creates. Imagine, therefore, if one is dealing with a patient who has allergies to wheat, corn, milk and yeast: there will be a different curve of symptomatology for each food, depending on the frequency with which it is eaten. Any relationship between food and symptoms will in these circumstances become far from obvious. I emphasize this point because many physicians believe that if food allergy is present, it will be obvious to all those concerned. It is partly this simplistic view of the subject which has led to its neglect.

The concept of masking is the single most important factor to grasp about the inter-relationship of food and asthma. It explains why so many asthmatic patients feel so bad first thing in the morning. Asthma patients often also feel worse if they happen to miss their breakfast, which normally contains one of the foods to which they are sensitive.

The concept of masking also explains why some foods eaten only on an occasional and intermittent basis are known by certain people to worsen their asthma. When I talk to asthmatic patients, a surprising number know that a certain occasionally eaten food may produce some worsening of their symptoms, although obviously other factors are operating, as avoidance of this food does not eliminate the problem. Patients often mention these observations to their chest physicians, who by and large ignore them.

Unfortunately, these observations, which were originally made 40 years ago, were ignored or misunderstood by the medical profession in general, but a full account of the concept was given in what is now the classic textbook on the subject: *Food Allergy* by Herbert J. Rinkel MD, Theron G. Randolph MD, and Michael Zeller MD, originally published in 1951. In this book the main basic concepts of food allergy are described in great detail.

Adaptation

Allergy represents the failure of an organism to adapt to its environment. Much human illness, therefore, stems from the inability of the human organism to adapt to new foods or chemicals brought into the environment, or to an overdosage of such items. The original concept of adaptation was first described by Hans Selye, an eminent physiologist working at McGill University in Montreal. In 1936 Selye's work was published in the journal *Nature*, entitled 'The General Adaptation Syndrome'. He described the Adaptation Syndrome as a characteristic set of events which could be produced by a wide range of harmful agents. He stated that experiments on rats showed that if the organism is severely damaged by acute non-specific harmful agents (such as exposure to cold, surgical injury, excessive muscular exercise, or intoxication with sub-lethal doses of diverse drugs), a typical syndrome appears, the symptoms of which are independent of the nature of the original damaging agent.

Selye described various stages of the development of this syndrome, which Dr. Theron Randolph soon realized were identical to the various facets he had observed in the development of allergy. The whole subject of masking, withdrawal symptomatology on avoidance of foods and the Rinkel Hyperacute Response fitted in exactly with Selye's observations of animals. The principles of adaptation and maladaptation are discussed much more extensively in Chapter 15. The concept of adaptation is dealt with quite brilliantly by Dr. Randolph in his book, *Allergies: Your Hidden Enemy*, co-authored by Ralph Moss.

Fixed and Cyclic Food Sensitivities

Food sensitivity can be divided into fixed food sensitivities and cyclic food sensitivities. A fixed food sensitivity is one which has probably been present since birth and will never go away. In other words, the individual may eat the food extremely rarely but will react adversely every time. He or she may avoid the food for 20 years and yet still react strongly to it if it is eaten. These fixed food sensitivities are comparatively rare and certainly account for less than 5 per cent of all food sensitivities. Fixed food sensitivities are nearly always the classic IgE-mediated type sensitivity described earlier (*see page 46*).

A food sensitivity which disappears within two years of complete avoidance of the food will generally be regarded as a cyclic food sensitivity. In a cyclic food sensitivity, the degree of reaction is related to the frequency of ingestion. One method of treatment other than desensitization (discussed in Chapter 13) is to avoid the food for a period of time, during which tolerance can develop. This time span usually varies between two and eight months, but by definition can extend up to two years. Usually, the stronger the symptoms that the food causes, the longer it takes for tolerance to develop. Tolerance can also, in exceptional circumstances, develop within two or three weeks; this is a potent source of problems when one is attempting to pinpoint food sensitivity by following an elimination diet, which may extend over a period of about five weeks.

Tolerance is, however, a fragile flower and can usually be maintained only if the individual eats the 'sensitive food' every five days. If the food is consumed more frequently than this, the sufferer nearly always starts to react to it again. I have seen patients who identify specific food sensitivities on an exclusion diet. Some months later they may eat the food again by mistake, but, having suffered no reaction, they conclude that their original observation was erroneous. Unless forewarned, they may then start to eat the food on a frequent basis, rapidly destroy their tolerance to it, and then start to react to it once more. These ideas about the development and subsequent maintenance of tolerance led to the development of what is known as the rotary diversified diet (*see page 69*).

Defining Allergy

Returning now to the food allergy component, it is probably at this point appropriate to clarify the term 'allergy'. In 1906 an Austrian physician called Clement von Pirquet coined the term from two Greek words which meant 'altered reactivity'. In other words, an allergy was a response to a substance which affected one individual but not another. Allergy therefore contrasts with toxicity. Toxicity affects everyone, though usually to varying degrees. Everyone is killed with hydrogen cyanide, but only some people react adversely to milk. About 1906 it was beginning to be realized that many illnesses were an interaction between environmental factors and susceptible individuals, and the term 'allergy' described this situation well.

The use or misuse of the term has caused the most amazing schisms among physicians working with patients who have adverse reactions to foods. Most immunologists assert that when von Pirquet coined the term 'allergy' he meant it to cover only those reactions in which a specific immunological (antigen-antibody) reaction could be determined. A colleague of von Pirquet, Dr. Doerr, in a paper published in 1909 quite definitely widened the use of the term to cover every form of altered reactivity, whether an underlying antigen-antibody reaction could be shown or not.

Close study of von Pirquet's writings shows that he realized that immune reactions and supersensitivities can be most closely related and often impossible to dissociate. He thus meant 'allergy' to be a term which would prejudice nothing and could cover reactions which had no known immunological basis. Because of this I use the word freely throughout this text.

The year 1925 was an historic one in the field of allergy, but for those physicians taking a wide view of allergy it was an 'infamous' one. Interest in food allergy had just started to grow, particularly in the US. However, in 1925 European and British allergists persuaded their American colleagues to restrict their definition of allergy to those mechanisms which could be explained by the antigen-antibody hypothesis. This, of course, made the field extremely 'scientific'. These reactions could be measured accurately in the laboratory and did not depend on the involvement of such unpredictable factors as actual patients and their own observations! The most eminent American immunologist of the day, Arthur F. Coca of Cornell University, fought strongly against this restrictive view, but most of his colleagues in the allergy profession went along with the new orthodoxy. The last 25 years, however, have seen the emergence of many physicians in North America, Great Britain and Australia who have reported countless cases of non-immunological allergy, and their work has re-challenged this narrow view of allergy. Many immunologically-orientated physicians have now come round to the same viewpoint, although there is still resistance from much of the immunological establishment.

Currently, therefore, the situation is that what is universally agreed to be food allergy is an immediate Type I reaction to food. It is character-ized by a rapid onset and is occasionally anaphylactic (a major collapse/shock reaction often accompanied by markedly reduced blood pressure) in nature. This type of reaction usually occurs in response to occasionally eaten exotic foods, and normally the patient is more than aware of the reaction. The problem is mediated by the immunoglobulin called IgE, and is easily demonstrated by a blood test called the RAST test. This is short for the Radioallergosorbent test, which measures levels of IgE antibodies in the blood in response to a specific substance, such as a food protein or a pollen.

The term 'food intolerance' is frequently used for all adverse reac-tions to food which have not been shown to be IgE mediated, and in the case of asthma virtually no foods which are implicated have been shown to cause IgE-mediated responses. There is a possible confusion here, since this definition of intolerance would include reactions mediated by other immunological mechanisms, such as IgG or immune complexes. Also, many food reactions 'look' immunological, in that they show intradermal skin reactions similar to the ones that would be observed in IgE-mediated allergy. Of course, there are also other ways in which human beings can react adversely to foods, which are definitely not allergy by any stretch of the imagination. These include:

- **Enzyme deficiencies** (for example, deficiencies of the enzyme lactase, whose function is to digest the milk sugar called lactose)
- **Toxicity** (certain foods can contain toxins, like the mould toxins sometimes found in grain that has been stored in damp conditions. These toxins [microtoxins] can produce symptoms in human beings)
- **Gut Dysbiosis (Candida)** (adverse reactions can, for example, be observed in response to the ingestion of sugar; the mechanism at work probably concerns the feeding of the various yeasts involved in this problem [*see Chapter 8*])

The Rotary Diversified Diet

The rotary diversified diet is one of the major tools in this field. People with minor allergy problems or with a sensitivity to only two or three foods will rarely need to use it. Sufferers who are adequately dealt with by desensitization will not usually need to use it. Those who have a Candida problem (*see Chapter 8*) need it less if their Candida is treated. Even if the patient does not go onto a formal rotary diet, it is advisable that the diet is varied as much as possible and that foods, especially those such as wheat, sugar and milk, are not repeated too frequently. In a classic rotary diversified diet, foods from certain food families are eaten on Day 1, others on Day 2, others on Day 3 and still others on Day 4; the whole procedure is then repeated. In other words, no foods are eaten on more than one day in every four. A comprehensive account of the rotary diversified diet is given in my book *Arthritis – Allergy, Nutrition and the Environment* (Thorsons, 1995). It is also described in many other books devoted to food allergy.

Allergy Tests

Elimination Diets

Elimination diets are undoubtedly the 'bench-mark' against which all other methods of testing should be measured. When going through an elimination diet it is possible to see in real life what is happening. If a patient has severe intrinsic type asthma, the improvement in the asthma can be attained by limiting the diet to a handful of safe foods for about six or seven days. If symptoms disappear on this regime, described in great detail in Chapter 11 (a low-risk diet), the patient knows where he or she stands. It is not in truth a great sacrifice to go on such a diet, as a few days of denial can change the future outlook from unmitigated pessimism to great optimism. The elimination diet has the virtue, also, that it is both simple and inexpensive. If there is no improvement shown on such a diet, then food sensitivity can be excluded as a possible cause of or contributor to a person's allergy.

The subsequent phase of re-introducing foods back into the diet may be just as simple, but it is fair to say that for someone with a large number of sensitivities, it can be very complicated and sometimes confusing.

Intradermal Provocative Skin Testing and Neutralization

This is a vast improvement on, and a refinement of, standard skin prick testing which has been used for many years in hospitals. There have been about 12 clinical trials which have established its validity and, used competently, it is a vital and extremely useful method of both diagnosis and treatment. About 15 clinics in the UK use the test extensively; in the US it is used currently by over 4,000 clinics. Without it we would not be able to help a large proportion of our more complicated patients. The test and concept is so important that I have devoted two chapters to the uses of this method (Chapters 12 and 13) and one (Chapter 14) to the trials validating its usage.

Prick Testing

This is a fairly useful test for inhalant allergies, but does not really help in the diagnosis of food allergy. It is this simple fact which has, in my opinion, held back, until recently, the development of interest in food allergy. The test involves placing a single drop of allergen extract on the inner forearm. A lancet is introduced through the drop of extract on the skin at an acute angle, and, having slightly penetrated the skin, is given a deliberate vertical lift before being removed. Responses to these tests are read after 10–20 minutes. Many of the tests can be performed within a few minutes of each other and the whole test is, therefore, both simple and quick to perform. Unhappily, it is not very effective because most patients with well-established food allergies will fail to react positively to this test. As we have become familiar with the intradermal provocative neutralizing test it has become apparent why prick tests are so useful for diagnosing inhalant allergies but useless for diagnosing food allergies. I have detailed these thoughts in Chapters 12 and 13.

Because prick tests have been used for so long, many people, including physicians, place unwarranted credence on their results. I have known patients with genuine food allergies who have been informed categorically that their allergies do not exist, purely on the basis of this test, and this can, therefore, do more harm than good. Dr. Keith Eaton of Reading published a trial showing that the prick test is of no value in diagnosing food allergy. As he put it, one is better off tossing a coin to determine food allergies than relying on this test.

RAST Test

As mentioned earlier, this is short for Radioallergosorbent Test and will only measure IgE-mediated allergy, which is relevant in the types of asthma related to allergies to dust, mites, moulds, etc., but is totally irrelevant in diagnosing food sensitivity, as almost all food sensitivity is not mediated by the immunoglobulin E. Hence, like prick testing for food sensitivity, the RAST test is a positive source of misinformation when it comes to the foods usually implicated in asthma.

Cytotoxic Testing

This is just about the most controversial of all tests for food allergy. There are a few physicians who enthusiastically promote cytotoxic testing, but the conventional allergy establishment and most members of the British Society for Allergy & Environmental Medicine are very sceptical about its value. It does, of course, have the superficial attraction of suggesting that countless food and chemical allergies can be diagnosed from a sample of blood. The term cytotoxic literally means 'having a toxic effect on cells'.

The blood sample is incubated on a microscope slide with a weak solution of suspected food allergen, and the effect on certain specific white cells is noted. In a positive test the polymorph leucocytes (one type of white cell) slow down, become rounded and also (in strongly positive cases) disintegrate. There is no doubt that this phenomenon occurs, but the interpretation of the results depends on the varying judgements of different technicians.

Scientific appraisals of the cytotoxic test show that food extracts do sometimes affect white blood cells in this way, and in a recent study under carefully controlled conditions, produced about 65 – 70 per cent accuracy. If this could be improved upon this test might be useful, but at present it gives so many wrong answers that it is of little value. Certainly, if this became a reliable test it could be extensively used by practitioners with little knowledge of allergy, and this would doubtless lead to a wider application of these principles in general medical practice.

Another big criticism of the cytotoxic test as it is currently used, and in my opinion a fair one, is that companies offering the test often do so directly to the public. Sometimes the test appears to uncover huge numbers of food sensitivities, and as a result some people may end up on a very harsh and possibly nutritionally inadequate diet, unsupervised by anyone with any knowledge of nutrition. Of course, such a situation arises partly because many physicians stubbornly refuse to have any involvement in the field of allergy medicine at all.

Applied Kinesiology

This method is particularly favoured by chiropractors, some of whom have taken an interest in the field of food allergy. Initially the practitioner establishes the patient's muscle strength and tone by observing how easily he or she can lift, for example, a 50-lb (23-kg) weight. An allergen is introduced, usually under the tongue, and muscle tone again measured. The theory is that an allergic reaction will weaken the muscle tone and that this can be detected by the practitioner. There may be something in this test, but there has been absolutely no scientific validation of it as yet. At the moment, as there are relatively well-validated alternatives in existence, I feel that they should be used in preference to applied kinesiology.

Radionics

Several people claim to be able to diagnose food allergies from hair samples. A pendulum is dangled over the hair sample: if it rotates in one way, allergy is indicated, if the pendulum rotates the opposite way, it is not. Although I accept that there are several very strange magnetic phenomena which we do not yet understand, this particular test stretches credibility to breaking point. I have had many patients who have seen me after they have been tested in this way, and the allergies that we have detected have borne little relationship to their hair test results.

The worst aspect of fringe tests such as cytotoxic testing, kinesiology and radionics is that many physicians who find the concept of food sensitivity dubious have seized upon these tests and their complete lack of scientific validation to criticize serious allergists, who do not use these tests anyway.

Sublingual Testing

When I was first interested in the subject of food allergy, I did quite a lot of tests using this method. The principle is the same as for the intradermal provocative test. Solutions are made up in nine separate concentrations with a 1-in-5 dilution factor between one strength and the next. The first strength is the strongest, the second is one-fifth weaker, and so on.

The technique consists of placing one measured drop of the food to be tested under the patient's tongue using a specially-designed dropper pipette. The area under the tongue is one of great absorbability, as the large sublingual veins are present there. The patient lies quietly on a couch and any resulting symptoms are noted. It is also usual to take the pulse and record the size of the pupils at intervals. If symptoms or other changes occur, successively weaker levels are administered until the symptoms are counteracted. A more elaborate description of this technique can be found in Richard Mackarness' book *Not All in the Mind* (Pan Books, 1976).

Sometimes, particularly when very soluble foodstuffs such as milk, tea, coffee, orange juice, etc. are introduced under the tongue, one can see dramatic and obvious reactions. With less soluble items, particularly items such as wheat and corn, reactions can easily fail to materialize despite the fact that the individual has a wheat or corn sensitivity. I cannot recall seeing anyone middle-aged who has had a dramatic reaction to wheat, corn, or any other cereal given sublingually.

The other disadvantage is that it is much more difficult to identify the neutralizing level when foods are tested in this way. This form of testing is inferior to intradermal provocation testing, as intradermal provocation testing has two pillars on which the assessment can be made — one represents the symptoms which are being induced or relieved, the other is the appearance of the wheal. These two facets complement each other, as the wheal changes normally correlate with the changes in symptom pattern. In some people, however, neither sublingual testing, nor even the intradermal testing will induce any symptoms whatsoever. With the intradermal testing one can at least observe the wheal response, but with sublingual testing one just has to record the test as negative, even if earlier testing proved there was a positive reaction.

Treatment for Food Allergies

There is one fairly well-established form of treatment for food allergy, and this is the **provocative intradermal neutralization** treatment, given either by injection or sublingual drops and validated by clinical trials (*see Chapter 14*).

The techniques and rationale of this approach are described in Chapters 12 and 13.

Less well validated is **enzyme potentiated desensitization**, developed by Dr. Len McEwen, who used to work at the Department of Allergy at St. Mary's Hospital in Paddington, London. Recently there has been more interest in this technique.

Nalcrom (sodium cromoglycate) has been shown in various clinical studies, like those produced by Dr. Derek Wraith and mentioned earlier in this chapter, to offer some protection against food sensitivities. It is taken by mouth prior to the ingestion of a known food sensitivity and it is supposed to stop the reaction by coating the allergy mediating (mast) cells and stopping them from reacting to presented allergens. Except for use to protect against an occasional meal containing specific allergies, I haven't found Nalcrom very helpful. Certainly, taken on a regular basis it is not really effective and is horrendously expensive to boot.

Conclusion

Food sensitivity is a major cause of asthma. Its role has been shamefully ignored by countless physicians whose only ambition is to suppress asthma symptoms by means of drugs. Chapter 3 clearly demonstrates the dangers of this course of action. As with any other illness, it is much better to remove the cause than to suppress the symptoms.

Chemical Sensitivity in Asthma

Chemical sensitivity is occupying an ever-increasing part in our thoughts when we consider what is initiating the asthma problem and what is perpetuating it.

Outdoor Pollutants

Although outdoor air pollution occupies the 'hot seat' in the popular imagination, it is now becoming much more obvious that indoor air pollution is more important, particularly in initiating the problem. Aside from both of these inhaled forms of chemical reactivity, there is no doubt that asthma can be provoked by chemicals in the food that we consume.

In Chapter 1 I mentioned the phenomenon of 'tolerance induction', a phenomenon which is almost certainly at the root of why some people develop asthma and others do not. It's also possible that there is another mechanism – for example, diesel smoke is believed to damage the lining of the lungs so that inhaled allergens pass through the barrier to the deeper tissues, activating the immune defences and triggering asthma. To return, however, to tolerance induction and to reiterate what I said in the introductory chapter, we all have an immune system which is similar to a defensive army. This army protects us from a huge range of assaults which our environment is inclined to throw at us. These include bacteria, viruses, fungi, yeasts and allergens. The prime function of the immune system is to distinguish between harmful and harmless invaders. Thus the immune system should act effectively against microbes which may well cause disease, but not react against harmless items such as pollens, dust mite and food molecules. The act of learning to distinguish and shrug off items that are harmless is called 'tolerance induction'. This process usually occurs when we first, as babies, meet a new allergen. In mice and rats it has been shown that an antigen (an item that is a potential allergen), if inhaled, automatically induces tolerance and prevents any production of the antibody Immunoglobulin E (IgE). It works through the good offices of some very special cells called T-suppressor cells, but unfortunately this system is not very well established in newborn rats or mice. Hence at this time they can be relatively easily sensitized by an inhaled antigen. This may well, for example, explain why human beings are more likely to develop hayfever if they are born just before the hayfever season. Of enormous importance, it has been shown that even in adult rats and mice the inhalation of certain chemicals can interfere with induction of tolerance.

High on the list of chemicals that can do this is the gas nitrogen dioxide, which is not only present in car exhaust fumes but is also spewed out from gas cookers and gas and oil boilers. These indoor air pollutants are discharged into our hermetically-sealed houses, where they remain in quite high concentrations for some time. Thus if an animal inhales a fair amount of nitrogen dioxide it can irritate the nose and the adjacent upper respiratory system. If this animal then inhales an antigen such as housedust mite, to which it has never previously been exposed, it will not become tolerant in the normal course of events.

Sulphur dioxide, which was such a major pollutant earlier this century, has also been shown in experimental animals to prevent tolerance induction, but most sulphur dioxide was encountered outside the house and was subject to dispersal in the atmosphere. These studies on tolerance induction were performed in mice and rats; and whether the same effect occurs in human beings is not known for certain, but, scientists think that it almost definitely is, as it is such a fundamental biological mechanism.

The evidence against nitrogen dioxide is now quite extensive. A 1993 case control study, amongst children aged 3 and 4 years old diagnosed for the first time with asthma, showed a striking association between the incidence of asthma and nitrogen dioxide as measured with a personal badge worn over a period of 24 hours.[1] Eminent commentators have suggested that nitrogen dioxide may act by decreasing the threshold of sensitization to allergen exposure.

Two 1994 reports in *The Lancet* showed that nitrogen dioxide alone[2] or in combination with sulphur dioxide[3] in concentrations usually encountered in daily life, enhance the adverse response to inhaled housedust mite in patients with mild asthma.

In a recent study, again published in *The Lancet*, even more evidence was gathered showing an 'association of respiratory symptoms in young adults with the use of domestic gas appliances'.[4] The study involved 15,000 adults in East Anglia. Women who reported that they mainly used gas for cooking were shown to have had an increased risk of severe asthma-like symptoms during the preceding 12 months. The differences were statistically significant. Women who used a gas stove or who had an open gas fire had reduced lung function (low forced expiratory volumes) and increased airways obstruction as compared with women who did not. These associations were not observed in men, probably because women cook more frequently than men.

In an American study published in *The Lancet*, cooking with a gas cooker generated concentrations of 200–400 parts per billion of nitrogen dioxide, with transient peaks as high as 1,000 parts per billion.[5] In a study in New Mexico[6] it was found that in 30 per cent of the two-weekly visits, children reported having been in the kitchen while meals were being cooked during the preceding 24 hours for an average of 20 minutes.

To contrast these levels of nitrogen dioxide, such as 400 to 1,000 parts per billion, it should be pointed out that outdoor levels of nitrogen dioxide of around 400 parts per billion are only encountered during very severe outdoor air pollution, which will only occur occasionally. Peak levels, for example of 382 to 423 parts per billion, were recorded during a severe pollution episode in London in December 1991. Thus the levels commonly occurring in the kitchen are only occasionally observed in outdoor air pollution. Thus it would appear likely that these increased levels of nitrogen dioxide, which can decrease tolerance induction, are also increasing the problem for those who already have asthma.[7]

There is a huge range of other chemicals, which are all hydrocarbons and derived from basic hydrocarbons like oil and gas, that have been categorically shown to provoke asthma. Once sensitization has occurred to one hydrocarbon, the problem is liable to occur with its other hydrocarbon cousins. These chemicals are often only inhaled intermittently and the resulting reaction is obvious in many cases to the patient.

In the study[8] carried out in New York at the Albert Einstein School of Medicine, patients were placed under a plastic canopy and exposed to four squirts of, for example, atomized cologne. Their forced expiratory volume fell between 18 and 58 per cent and they complained of chest tightening and wheezing within one to two minutes of exposure. Of the 60 asthmatic patients surveyed, 57 complained of respiratory reactions with exposure to 'common odours'. The findings were:

Insecticides	85% reacted
Household cleaners	78% reacted
Cigarette smoke	75% reacted
Perfumes and cologne	72% reacted
Fresh paint	73% reacted
Car exhaust fumes	60% reacted
Cooking smells	37% reacted

Sweden has contributed to our knowledge of this subject. In 1995, a study relating asthmatic symptoms, volatile organic compounds, formaldehyde, and carbon dioxide was published in the *Journal of Occupational & Environmental Medicine*.[9] The study concluded that symptoms related to asthma were more common in dwellings with housedust mites and visible signs of dampness or microbial growth in the building. Significant relationships were also found between nocturnal breathlessness and the presence of wall-to-wall carpets and indoor concentrations of carbon dioxide, formaldehyde, and volatile organic compounds (formaldehyde is extensively used in wool carpets, for example). The researchers concluded that these volatile organic compounds and formaldehyde are likely to cause asthmatic symptoms, and that there was a need to increase the outdoor air supply to many dwellings and reduce the amount of dampness and the use of wall-to-wall carpeting.

There is absolutely no doubt that smoking, either active or passive, is a very major cause of asthma. Cigarette smoke is a potent mixture of a whole range of chemicals, and very many asthmatics are aware that they will wheeze if exposed to other people's cigarette smoke. It is my opinion that any asthmatic who actively smokes cigarettes is mad, although I do accept that it is often very hard for an addicted cigarette smoker to 'kick' the habit. There have been countless studies linking asthma and cigarette smoke and also, quite recently, linking cigarette smoke with infant cot deaths.

In 1988, Stankus *et al*.[10] studied 21 asthmatics, 19 of whom were atopic, who complained of wheezing when exposed to cigarette smoke. Seven of the 21 experienced significant reductions in their ability to perform pulmonary function tests when exposed to cigarette smoke for two hours. Of interest was the finding that the other 14 asthmatics, who claimed that they were sensitive to cigarette smoke, did *not* experience bronchospasm with challenge testing. Very probably they would have done so had they been in the de-adapted state (that is, if they had avoided exposure for about five days before the challenge test). This masking phenomena applies equally to chemical sensitivity as it does to food sensitivity.

In a British study from St. George's Hospital Medical School in London, 1996,[11] studying concurrently various factors affecting asthmatics up to the age of 33, two of the major conclusions were that the incidence of asthma in the age group 17–33 was strongly associated with active cigarette smoking and a history of hayfever. Furthermore, relapse by the age of 33 after prolonged remission of childhood wheezing was more common amongst current smokers and atopic subjects. Thus, the case against cigarette smoking in relation to asthma is very strong, and I will not labour this point any longer.

> At the core of the chemical sensitivity problem is the conundrum that there is no doubt at all that diesel fumes, petrol fumes, ozone and sulphur dioxide emissions can all be shown to precipitate an attack of asthma. Despite this, in the Isle of Skye, perhaps the least polluted part of the United Kingdom, it has been shown that there is a higher rate of asthma than in many industrial cities like Aberdeen.[12]

The most spectacular example of outdoor air pollution and its effect on human beings was the notorious winter smog of 1952 that killed approximately 4,000 Londoners. Not all of those who died were asthmatic, but a lot were. What happened in this was that large amounts of smoke from coal fires entered the atmosphere at the same time as there was a major winter anti-cyclone. This anti-cyclone settled over London on December 5th 1952 and preceded a rare period of very calm non-windy weather. Temperature inversion, which consists of a cold layer of air at ground level enveloped by a zone of warmer air higher up, prevented the air from circulating. This led to the build-up of emissions from low-lying industrial and domestic chimneys. These trapped emissions combined with moisture in the cold air to form a lethal fog of acid vapour and black smoke.

In the winter of 1909, Glasgow experienced two severe smogs, followed by another in 1929. All of these events were followed by an increase in mortality. In December 1930, after five days of polluted fog, approximately 60 people died in the Belgian industrial Meuse Valley. There have been several other examples of this phenomenon in various parts of the industrial world.

The UK's Clean Air Act made this type of pollution a thing of the past, but nowadays virtually all industrial cities spend the summer draped in a photochemical haze caused by the effect of sunlight on the products of vehicle exhaust systems. Sunlight catalyses the conversion of vehicle exhaust emissions such as nitrogen dioxide, carbon monoxide, other hydrocarbons and various particulates with some low-level industrial pollutants, to produce ozone.

Numerous studies have shown that ozone can increase bronchial responsiveness and impair lung function in a proportion of normal subjects and in people with asthma. In particular, one study of 3,914 non-smoking Californian 7th Day Adventists showed a relationship between the development of new cases of asthma in men between 1977 and 1987 and ambient concentrations of ozone.[13]

A German study of the effect of road traffic on children in Munich also showed that high volumes of road traffic do lead to diminished forced expiratory flow and increased respiratory symptoms in children.[14]

Yet, despite the fact that exposure to exhaust fumes, ozone and sulphur dioxide can be shown to produce asthmatic attacks, I agree with the statement of the Committee on the Medical Effects of Air Pollutants, set up by the British Government to examine the links between asthma and air pollution. They concluded that daily fluctuations in the levels of air pollution do correlate with hospital admissions and symptoms, but that this accounts for less than 5 per cent of the total number of episodes of asthma. The overall conclusion of their report was that the effect of outdoor air pollution on asthma was small. Indeed, the effect was almost certain to be small when one considers the results of the trial which showed that the incidence of asthma on the Isle of Skye, arguably the area of least outdoor air pollution in the whole of the United Kingdom, was higher than that of industrial cities like Aberdeen.

The national average for reported asthma is around 11 per cent. In Skye the figure was 17 per cent. In addition the prevalence of some degree of wheeze was actually 28 per cent, and bronchospasm (wheeze after exercise) was found to be 30 per cent.[15] There is no industrial outdoor pollution in Skye, and very few cars. The only man-made outdoor pollution on the whole island would be the smoke from some household fires, which would be rapidly dispersed by the winds so prevalent in that location. This study is in fact supported by other studies showing little causal relationship between outdoor chemical pollution and asthma. A study published in 1994[16] compared the incidence of asthma in Munich and Leipzig. Before the fall of the Berlin Wall there was horrific outdoor pollution in Leipzig. The amount of sulphur dioxide was 30 times worse than in Munich, and particulate matter in the air was 10 times worse. Despite all this, asthma was more common in Munich.

Thus, while we are fairly sure that outdoor chemical pollution can make asthma worse, it does not look as if it is important in the original induction of the process, and as stated earlier it is beginning to look as if indoor air pollution is the biggest culprit in this story. There has been a marked increase in chemical pollution over the past 30 years, compounded by the hermetic sealing of homes and hence also increased exposure to the housedust mite. It would certainly be very interesting to return to the Isle of Skye and try to correlate the incidence of asthma there with various types of indoor air pollution. Although there is no natural gas on the island there is fairly extensive use of calor gas for heating and cooking, and of oil and coal fires. As the island is a fairly cold place to live, one would imagine that the hermetic sealing would be pretty good and it would be possible that indoor air pollution could be worse on this island than in the average city. Skye would in fact be a wonderful laboratory to study indoor air pollution divorced from the effect of outdoor air pollution.

Indoor Air Pollution

The effect of outdoor air pollution, which is often very obvious to the asthma sufferer, contrasts with the effect of indoor air pollution which is usually more continuous, more hidden, more subtle and more significant. Many hydrocarbon-sensitive people are aware of the fact that intermittently presented hydrocarbons such as perfumes, petrol fumes, nail varnish, printer's ink and dry-cleaning fluids are able to induce symptoms of one sort or another, but these individuals are almost always ignorant of the fact that more continuously inhaled chemicals may be playing a part in their problems. The more continuously inhaled chemicals include:

- domestic gas from gas cookers, gas fires and gas central heating
- calor gas
- formaldehyde
- trichlorethylene
- phenol
- xylene
- toluene
- cigarette smoking.

There are several others, but these just happen to be amongst the more prevalent.

Because of its relative cheapness, natural gas is present in a very high proportion of British homes, both for central heating and for cooking. Reactions to gas are probably more frequently implicated in asthma than any other single chemical, but if an oil-fired central heating boiler is situated within the confines of the house, it can cause similar problems.

Formaldehyde is another major problem. In the 1970s and 1980s there was a vogue for cavity wall insulation with urea formaldehyde foam, and when the dangers of it became realized in the UK it was quietly dropped and replaced by other methods. In the US it created a huge scandal, and whole housing estates had to be abandoned because amongst the occupants there developed a very high incidence of asthma, rhinitis, persistent coughs, skin rashes and so forth. In one study, houses with urea foam formaldehyde had a mean average formaldehyde level of 0.12 parts per million, while an average house without this insulation had a mean level of 0.03 parts per million. In other words the formaldehyde insulation quadrupled the normal level. However, in highly energy efficient homes, even without urea foam formaldehyde insulation, levels of 0.10 parts per million were shown because the tightening of the insulation ensured the retention of formaldehyde out-gassed from other products.

Typical readings of formaldehyde in various environments are as follows:

	Parts per million
Normal house	0.03
Energy efficient house	0.10
House with urea formaldehyde cavity wall insulation	0.12
Mobile home	0.40
Office buildings	0.44
Hospitals	0.55
Shopping malls	1.50
Biological laboratory	8.50

The hospital reading of 0.55 parts per million is quite disgraceful in an institution which is supposed to restore health, and it is one reason why so many chemically sensitive patients feel so ill whenever they go to hospital. The high reading in biological laboratories is presumably because of the use of formalin (a solution of formaldehyde and water) to preserve specimens for dissection.

In cases where people have problems with formaldehyde it can be very difficult to exclude it from the house, as it out-gasses from carpets (particularly wool), mattresses, foam cushions, ceiling tiles, plaster-board, adhesives, cleaning solutions, fabrics, cigarette smoke and air fresheners. Carpets, in particular, are a concoction of chemicals, and most wool carpets contain formaldehyde, toluene, xylene, benzene, tetrachlorethylene, methyl'natpthalene, pthalates and styrene. These chemicals continue to out-gas for many years after the carpet is laid, particularly when the room is hot.

Trichlorethelene is another major contaminant of buildings and is used in:

- carpet shampoo
- dry-cleaning fluid (as used to clean clothes)
- floor polish
- photocopying machines
- furniture glues
- various machine oils and oil solvents.

Phenol is the chemical which is given off when plastics out-gas. The softer the plastic and the greater the heat, the faster the plastic out-gasses. Department stores, where there are many soft plastic coverings, have a lot of this odour, particularly when it is warm. Phenol is a toxic benzene derivative and is the old carbolic acid that has been used so extensively in hospitals. Phenol was used for a long time in many allergy extracts, but we have endeavoured to remove it from the range that we use at my clinic, because the last thing we wish to do is to add to a patient's chemical load.

Xylene is also a relative of benzene, and benzene is a known carcinogen, and this also out-gasses from many products, such as carpets.

Toluene is a solvent which out-gasses from products such as paint, especially gloss paint. Patients who notice that gloss paint when first applied makes them wheeze, are usually reacting to the toluene component.

Most of these chemicals have been implicated in patients with asthma at one time or another, at my clinic and at those of my colleagues.

Chemicals in Food

Practically any chemical used in food production can be implicated in asthma. Physicians who look into what is causing asthma have observed asthmatic reactions to a huge range of ingested chemicals in some of their patients. I emphasize *some* in that a great number of them have no reactions to chemicals at all and are purely reacting to other items such as housedust mite. Some of these chemical reactions have been examined in formal clinical studies published in medical journals. For example, Dr. B.J. Franklin of Kings College Hospital, London,[17] noted that of 272 patients with asthma 11 per cent noted exacerbations occurring after ingestion of orange drinks. Fourteen patients who noticed such exacerbations were given provocation tests by drinking, on separate occasions, solutions of sulphur dioxide, sodium benzoate and tartrazine, which are present in orange drinks. Eight reacted to sulphur dioxide, with a fall in their forced expiratory volumes, four to sodium benzoate and one to tartrazine. Four did not react to any of these chemicals. These three chemicals are used widely throughout the food industry. Sulphur dioxide, for example, is used in the production of various dried foods such as raisins, and is also used to stop pre-cut potato chips from browning at the edges. Other uses are to prevent vegetable spoilage in salad bars and stopping the fermentation process in the production of wines and beers. Sulphite sensitivity has also been reported in asthma in several other studies.[18]

Another chemical in food which has been shown to produce asthma is monosodium glutamate.[19] All these results have been demonstrated in blind placebo controlled challenges.

Although not demonstrated formally, many allergists have observed asthmatic reactions to:

- insecticides and pesticides
- ethylene gas, used to ripen bananas
- paraffin wax, used to coat cucumbers, apples and green peppers to improve their appearance and keep them edible for a longer period of time.

I have touched only briefly on this subject. It is covered in much greater detail in Dr. Theron Randolph's book *Human Ecology and Susceptibility to the Chemical Environment* (Charles C. Thomas), which was the first book published on this subject. There is also extensive coverage in the book *Allergies: Your Hidden Enemy* (Thorsons), again by Dr. Randolph but written in collaboration with R. W. Moss, Ph.D. Dr. Richard Mackarness has devoted a whole book to the subject *Chemical Victims* (Pan). More recently, in 1990, Dr. Sherry Rogers, the eminent American Environmental Physician, gave a vivid and entertaining account of this whole problem in her book *Tired or Toxic* (Prestige Publishing). I would recommend this book to anyone who wishes to look further into this subject. In 1991 Professor Nicholas Ashford, of the Massachusetts Institute of Technology and the Environmental Protection Agency, combined with Professor Claudia Miller, of the University of Texas, to produce an account of this problem from a highly academic viewpoint. Their book was entitled *Chemical Exposures – Low Levels and High Stakes* (Van Nostrand Reinhold). Their book is indicative of an increasingly high level of debate in the US on the subject of chemical sensitivity. For example, a workshop on health risks from exposure to common indoor household products in allergic or chemically diseased persons was held by the National Academy of Sciences in July 1987. It recommended an 18-month study to address the 15 per cent of the American population who have an increased sensitivity to chemicals commonly found in household products, which placed them at an increased risk of disease. In 1989 the National Academy of Sciences convened a panel to examine the inter-relationships of toxic exposure and immune response, and there are many other studies of a similar nature going on to this day.

Within the past few years Professor W.J. Rea, who is Head of the Environmental Health Centre in Dallas, has produced volumes 1–4 of the work entitled *Chemical Sensitivity* (Lewis Publishers). This truly epic work, comprising approximately 2,000 pages, is without doubt the definitive statement on this complex and totally fascinating subject.

Diagnosing the Problem

Many readers may wonder at this point how a physician can possibly sort out all the possible culprits on an out-patient basis. A patient's medical history can usually excite the allergist's suspicions. Intradermal provocative skin testing with synthetic ethanol, natural gas exhaust extracts, formaldehyde, phenol, toluene (the major constituent of gloss paint), trichloroethylene, etc. is also vital. If a positive skin reaction to any of these is obtained, especially if the strongest dose engenders symptoms, suspicion obviously increases. If these symptoms can be turned off or 'relieved' by finding a weaker neutralizing dose of that chemical, the strong suspicion amounts to certainty. If the symptoms of asthma can be turned on by one concentration of a chemical and turned off by another, it is very persuasive evidence that that chemical is relevant to that patient's problems.

The Environmental Control Unit

Rarely, asthma is too complex to sort out with the type of outpatient measures mentioned above, and the sufferer may need to enter an environmental control unit. This is an in-patient clinic made from materials such as glass, metal, concrete, ceramic tile, porcelainized steel, etc., which do not out-gas. Air is fed into the unit through positive pressure filtration so that most potential chemical and biological inhalant allergens are filtered out. While in the unit a patient may fast for a few days to check that he or she is not ingesting any allergens.

In the US there are several of these units, but in the UK at the time of writing there is only one: the Airedale Allergy Centre in Airedale, near Keighley in North Yorkshire, which is run by Dr. Jonathan Maberly. This unit and others like it are particularly suitable for people with very complex food and inhalant sensitivities. After symptom clearance, patients are first challenged with organic foods and later with inhaled substances. The inhalant tests are done in 'sniff boxes' which are rather like telephone booths. Patients, while under observation, are exposed to chemicals in these booths. They do not know the precise nature of the chemicals to which they are being exposed, but later the results of these tests are discussed with them. People with certain chemical sensitivities, such as to gas, may have to have changes made to their homes; while some may have to take neutralizing drops or injections, and some may have to live off organic food and bottled spring waters.

There are, therefore, three ways of diagnosing chemical sensitivity:

1. History
2. Intradermal skin testing
3. 'Sniff boxes' within an environmental control unit.

The last tends to be needed only in the most extreme cases.

Until several years ago, dealing with chemical sensitivity consisted of identifying the problem followed by avoidance or densitization. In the case of continually inhaled allergens, avoidance was clearly the most effective strategy. The removal of gas appliances remains the most common thing that we have to recommend, but it is never done before the patient has tried turning off his or her appliances on a trial basis.

Stripping formaldehyde or plastic out of certain modern houses can be quite a formidable task, but there is a Formaldehyde Spot Test developed by Dr. Sherry Rogers in the US. A spot of this diagnostic reagent can be applied to suspicious fittings, and if the test is positive the source of formaldehyde is identified.

Neutralization works well for occasional contacts like petrol and diesel fumes, but only gives temporary protection and never really desensitizes the patient to those chemicals.

Toxicity and Chemical Sensitivity

The biggest advance in the past few years is the realization that toxicity and chemical sensitivity are really variations on a theme. For a long time the difference between toxicity and chemical sensitivity was thought to be quite distinct. However, in occupational medicine it is now realized that there is no absolutely safe level of chemical exposure. Some people will only respond adversely to large doses of chemicals, some to medium and some to extremely minor doses. There is, therefore, a continuum, and people who are thought of as chemically sensitive have, in effect, weak defences against these chemicals.

This means we must look to our detoxification system. Most people will be familiar with their respiratory systems, their cardio-vascular systems, their alimentary systems, urinary systems, musculo-skeletal systems and their nervous systems. Also, in the past few years most will have learned that they have an immune system — a defence against infection. However, until recently most people have not heard of the detoxification system. When, eventually, physicians realize its importance to current medicine it will change medicine for ever, bringing it into a new era where the suppression of symptoms will be supplanted by the identification of the causes of disease.

The process of detoxification is the way by which human beings deal with ingested chemicals and render them less toxic. Such foreign chemicals, known as **xenobiotics**, can be inhaled, eaten or absorbed through the skin. These chemicals are detoxified by various enzyme and other systems which change them to harmless chemicals which are excreted either in the urine or via the bile duct into the gut.

In recent years the use of the term detoxification has been questioned by some scientists, as occasionally the system malfunctions so severely that the harmful chemicals can be made more toxic, not less so. Hence, some people prefer the term **biotransformation**, as it does not imply that the process is universally beneficial.

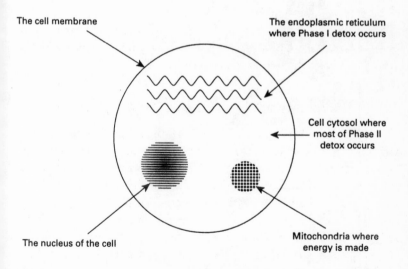

Figure 16 The Human Cell

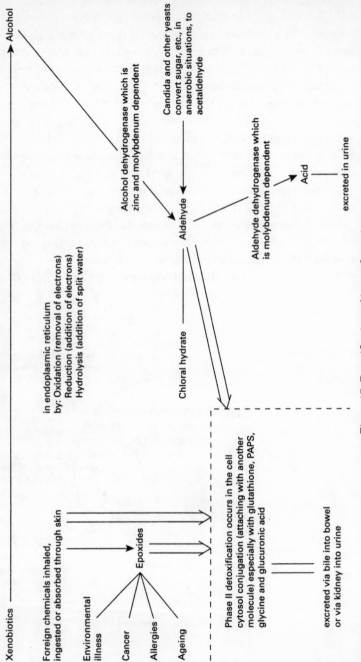

Figure 17 Detoxification or biotransformation

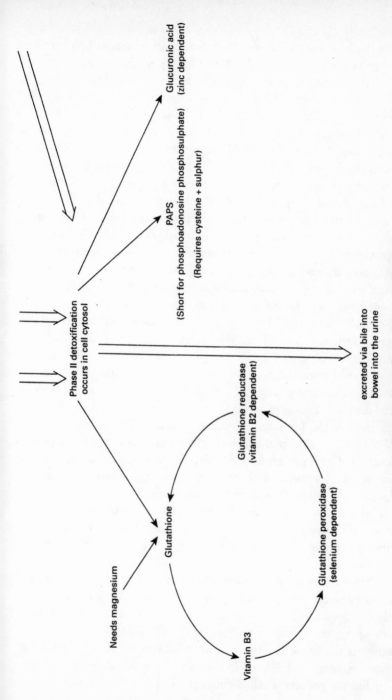

Figure 18 Phase II – Detoxification or biotransformation

Figures 16, 17 and 18 show simplified maps of the human cell and the main pathways of the detox or biotransformation system. Another name for this main system is the P450 cytochrome system. In the human cell diagram (Figure 16) one can see the nucleus, the cell membrane, the endoplasmic reticulum and the substance of the cell, which is called cytosol. On the Phase I map (Figure 17), one can follow the main stages of the detoxification process. The Phase I mechanism is represented by single lines and is the preferred mechanism. The Phase II, or back-up system is depicted by double lines. The Phase I system occurs in the endoplasmic reticulum, which is the wavy set of membranes shown in Figure 16 and, as you can see, the foreign chemical is first of all subjected to three processes of oxidation, reduction and hydrolysis, which convert the chemical into an alcohol. This alcohol is then acted upon by an enzyme called alcohol dehydrogenase which converts it into an aldehyde, such as acetaldehyde. This enzyme requires adequate amounts of zinc and molybdenum to function properly. Hence we can immediately see the influence of nutrition on our ability to handle chemicals. The acetaldehyde, in turn, is then converted by acetaldehyde dehydrogenase to an acid which is excreted in the urine. This hydrogenase enzyme is dependent for its proper function on molybdenum. It can be seen from the diagram that Candida fermentation in the gut produces excessive amounts of acetaldehyde which then tends to overload the Phase I detox pathway. When a lot of acetaldehyde is produced, this leads to the formation of chloral hydrate. Chloral hydrate is the 'Mickey Finn' (a drop of which knocks people out in the old detective novels) and with this excessive production of acetaldehyde one can see why so many patients with chemical sensitivity complain of feeling 'spaced out', 'fatigued' or 'downright unconscious'.

This tie-up with the Candida yeast problem, about which I go into great detail in Chapter 8, also explains the observation that many patients improve their chemical sensitivity when their Candida problem is treated.

When we were designed, someone clearly recognized that in the 20th century we were going to surround ourselves with about 60,000 chemicals that we had never met before, and considered that we needed a back-up system to cope with this huge load. This back-up system is known as the Phase II detox system and it comes into play when the Phase I system is overloaded. In Figure 18 it is represented by a double line, and the process is called **conjugation** and occurs in the **cytosol** part of each cell. Conjugation means adding on, and in this case the nutrients involved in conjugation are amino acids, which are the building blocks of proteins. Glutathione is the main conjugator of the Phase II detox system and is a tripetide consisting of three amino acids – glutamic acid, cysteine and glyceine. Each molecule of chemical needs one molecule of glutathione to detoxify it, and so chemically-sensitive patients show almost universal reduction in glutathione.

The trace mineral magnesium is absolutely vital for glutathione synthesis, and this is just one role that it plays in the chemical sensitivity story. Magnesium, in fact, is involved in nearly 300 different enzyme systems, and is a necessary co-factor for many of these reactions. Glutathione has to be constantly recycled, and the main parts of this recycling are represented in the Phase II diagram. As Figure 18 shows, Vitamin B_3, glutathione peroxidase (selenium dependent) and glutathione reductase (vitamin B_2 dependent) are major players in this process. Other chemicals that are needed in the process are PAPS (which is short for phosphoadenosine phosphosulphate) and glucuronic acid (zinc dependent).

Epoxidation

So, what happens when both the Phase I and the back-up Phase II mechanisms become overloaded? It is at this point that life starts to get serious because the whole chemistry shifts to the production of other metabolites called **epoxides** (as shown in Figure 17).

These chemicals are very reactive and unstable and attack cell membranes, which in turn lead to the symptoms of environmental illness and poisoning of the immune system. These epoxides can also initiate the changes leading to accelerated ageing, cancer and mutagenesis (undesirable changes in the genetic code). Thus, the formation of epoxides is the chemical reaction that immediately precedes the formation of symptoms, and it occurs because of overload of the Phase I and Phase II detox pathways. The formation of chloral hydrate, also shown in Figure 17, is another way in which symptoms can be triggered, and in the case of chloral hydrate they are usually of fatigue, a feeling of being 'spaced out' and poor concentration.

I am sorry for all the biochemistry, but there is really no other way to explain how detoxification works and how important nutrition is in correcting chemical sensitivity. We find that correcting nutritional deficiencies in these circumstances makes a tremendous difference, unless the enzyme pathways have been irreversibly damaged by huge and constant exposure to certain chemicals.

The nutrients that are in short supply vary a lot from patient to patient, and we make extensive use of a major nutritional biochemistry laboratory, The Biolab Medical Unit in London. This is a physician referral laboratory only. There are very few of these laboratories in the world, and they are equipped with modern high-technology equipment such as atomic absorption photo-spectrometers and liquid phase gas chromatographs.

Magnesium status can be assessed by a red blood cell magnesium test, a sweat test or a magnesium retention test.

Zinc status can best be measured by a leucocyte (white blood cell) zinc test or a sweat test.

Selenium status is best measured by a red blood cell selenium test or a test for the enzyme glutathione peroxidase. Low amounts of this particular enzyme indicate selenium deficiency, as it is totally dependent on adequate amounts of selenium.

Molybdenum status is a bit more difficult to estimate, but it is essential for the production of the enzyme sulphite oxidase, which metabolizes sulphites. A large amount of sulphite in the urine would indicate that this enzyme is not doing its stuff, and that the patient is deficient in molybdenum.

Levels of Vitamin B$_3$ and B$_2$ are also possible to measure and are important in chemical sensitivity.

Glutathione status can also be measured, but as the test is quite expensive and as it is nearly always depressed in patients with chemical sensitivity, I usually make the assumption that there is a reduced level.

Any of these trace minerals or vitamins should be supplemented if they are found to be depressed. Glutathione complex and magnesium are perhaps the most frequently useful supplements in treating chemical sensitivity.

To summarize the chemical sensitivity problem:

- It is very important in a proportion of sufferers from asthma.
- It is not surprising that some human beings should have problems with chemicals. Living organisms can adapt to many changes in their environment, but this adaptation often takes many generations and

tends not to be universal. Since the Second World War, in particular, there has been an enormous explosion in newly discovered chemicals, and the chemical industry has now quite revolutionized modern life. In Europe and the US billions of pounds of chemicals are produced annually, and over 25,000 different chemicals are in common use in the UK alone. Many of these chemicals find their way into our bodies. The testing of these chemicals is hardly comprehensive, and certainly takes no account of people who may be highly susceptible. As yet, no one has any idea of the cumulative effect of all these chemicals, and this is the most worrying aspect of the whole problem. Nobody knows how these individual chemicals interact within the confines of the human frame. The 20th century has been rightly described as an enormous, uncontrolled experiment on the human race.

- There are techniques now available for identifying chemical sensitivity.
- Having identified the problem, the best way to make a dramatic difference in the short term, is to avoid any chemical substances to which there is continual exposure, and to thus reduce the total load. Intermittent exposure can be dealt with by neutralizing drops.
- The long-term solution lies in the correction of nutritional deficiencies that underlie the chemical sensitivity, or the treatment of intestinal candidiasis, but it is still important to have a drastic reduction in the level of continuous exposure to chemicals.

There is extensive evidence that during the last 40 years we have had a diminished intake of certain major nutrients (*see Chapter 9*). At the same time there has been a massive increase in the amount of chemicals that we inhale and that we eat. So, just at the time we need our detox system to be functioning at its very best to deal with this pollutant overload, we are denying our enzyme systems the nutrients they need to carry out this task.

Without doubt, this is one of the major causes of the asthma epidemic.

Candida Hypersensitivity and Asthma

Most people have heard of an infection called thrush. Many women, for example, are plagued with recurring vaginal thrush. Oral thrush is well known in babies and in people who use Becotide or other steroid inhalers for asthma. Penile thrush is well recognized as a problem occurring in men. It is also well recognized that, if a patient's immune system becomes seriously compromised as a result of the use of immunosuppressive drugs, for example in the treatment of leukaemia, a serious generalized systemic thrush infection can occur, which can be fatal. Huge doses of anti-fungal drugs have to be given in such cases, often as a life-saving measure. The immunosuppressive drugs markedly weaken the patient's resistance to organisms such as thrush, which has always been known to be very much an opportunistic organism. In other words, when the host's defences are down, it can proliferate unchecked.

The medical term for thrush is Candida. The most prevalent strain of Candida is *Candida albicans*, probably the one strain that is most capable of inducing illness. There is another name for Candida, and that is Monilia. For the rest of this chapter I will refer to this problem as Candida.

All the above is well-received wisdom in the medical fraternity. What now follows, although there is a lot of evidence for it, is not. However, there are quite a number of clinical papers in respectable medical journals that have demonstrated a role for Candida in various disease processes; some of these will be mentioned later in this chapter. A perusal of the bookshelves in most healthfood shops will reveal a whole host of titles referring to Candida albicans: *The Yeast Connection*; *The Yeast Syndrome*; *Is Yeast Your Problem?* and so forth. Women's magazines, the health pages of national daily newspapers, and countless other publications are full of advice regarding the diagnosis and treatment of the Candida problem. Many thousands of patients have reported highly satisfactory recoveries from various chronic ailments which had previously been resistant to other treatments.

Thus, there are two views of the role of Candida in human illness: (1) the conventional view, suggesting that it has a limited role; and (2) the more expanded view, suggesting it has a huge role and is a factor in many disease processes, including, for example, eczema, urticaria, acne, psoriasis, irritable bowel syndrome, Crohn's disease, migraine, rheumatoid arthritis, endometriosis and several other conditions. Importantly, for those who are interested in asthma there is evidence that it plays a role in this condition as well.

There are, for example, papers describing a role for Candida in eczema, urticaria and psoriasis.[1] Evidence for its role in rheumatoid arthritis can be found in my book, *Arthritis – Allergy, Nutrition and the Environment*. Its role in migraine is discussed in my book, *The Migraine Revolution*.

Thus, Candida albicans seems to be a basic cause of a huge number of chronic disease processes, in the same way as are food sensitivity, chemical sensitivity, biological inhalant sensitivity and nutritional deficiencies. Thus, eczema, for example, can be shown in some cases to result from food sensitivity,[2] dust mite sensitivity[3] and Candida albicans.[4]

My first introduction to this expanded view of the role of Candida was through a presentation by Dr. Orion Truss at the 15th Advanced Seminar of the American Academy of Environmental Medicine in Atlanta, Georgia in 1982. Like most very important discoveries in medicine, this was made totally by accident. It sprang from the observation by a patient that, when she was given a neutralizing dose of Candida albicans (for a persistent skin infection), her depressive symptomatology disappeared for a few hours, for the first time for several years. The same effect occurred when she was given a further dose a few hours later. Subsequently, Dr. Truss treated her with high doses of anti-fungal drugs, combined with a yeast-free, sugar-free diet – thus curing her depression.

Dr. Truss at this time realized that the role of these organisms in human illness was much wider that he had previously thought and, having spent several years researching the role of Candida in human illness, he reported his observations in three separate papers in the *Journal of Orthomolecular Medicine*.[5] These papers did not make a great impact on the medical profession in general, mostly I think because physicians could not perceive how these findings could fit in with their existing knowledge and medical practice. However, physicians in the environmental field, who were looking at illness purely in terms of cause and effect, knew that they had been missing a major cause of illness, and so this work fell on much more receptive ears.

I have called this chapter Candida Hypersensitivity as it is quite clear that the problem does not entirely relate to the quantity of Candida found in each individual patient. Some patients clearly are riddled with the organism, but many appear to have average, or less than average, quantities within their gut.

Yet, despite this, their symptoms seem to respond brilliantly to the treatment. Many patients have a marked skin reaction to tests with dilute extracts of Candida albicans, suggesting an immune response rather than a simple infection.

Because of the lack of correlation between the quantity of Candida within the gut and symptoms, some researchers have even wondered whether Candida itself is actually involved, and whether the relief of symptoms brought about by anti-fungal treatment is due to a therapeutic effect other than the killing off of the Candida. Personally, I think this is unlikely, as these drugs vary considerably in their structure and mode of action, and because patients' skin responses seem to confirm with a hypersensitivity response.

At this point I should point out that in my experience Candida hypersensitivity plays a fairly small role in causing asthma, probably just under 10 per cent. This observation concurs with researchers who have published papers relating to this connection. In Chapter 4, I discussed the case history of a woman in whom Candida played a large but not exclusive role in the causation of her asthma.

There have been about four good clinical trials demonstrating a clear link between Candida and asthma.

In 1966, many years before Dr. Orion Truss made his discoveries (in the late 1970s), Itkin and Dennis from Denver, Colorado, published a major extensive and highly persuasive paper linking Candida and asthma.[6] The paper started with a statement that it is a scientific aim of the allergist to reduce the number of patients who must be classified as suffering from 'asthma of unknown origin' – clearly two men after my own heart. Eighty one in-patients were challenged quantitatively with aerosols of saline, 30 per cent glycerine, extracts of common inhalant allergens, and an extract of Candida albicans. The results of these challenges showed that Candida hypersensitivity is a factor of importance in some patients with severe asthma. The immediate skin response to a 1-in-1000 extract of Candida, and the reaction of the bronchial tree to other mould extracts, were correlated, with a positive bronchial reaction to Candida albicans extract in the patients studied.

In summary, the authors state that this study provides adequate documentation that Candida albicans is an atopic allergen, capable of evoking asthmatic response in suitable subjects. This effect appears to be clearly separate from any non-specific irritation or toxic effect, and from the pathogenic qualities of the Candida organism.

In 1987, Gumowski and Girard published a study in the *Annals of Allergy*[7] entitled, 'Chronic Asthma and Rhinitis due to Candida albicans, Epidermophyton, and Trichophyton'. Epidermophyton and trichophyton are two other yeast organisms frequently coexisting with Candida albicans. In the summary, they state that during the years 1982–83, all cases of chronic asthma exhibiting a positive skin test to Candida, trichophyton or epidermophyton were selected for the study. Sixty of these cases were of asthma and 75 were of rhinitis. All went through various nasal and bronchial provocation tests with the specific antigens identified. An immediate response was discovered in 91 cases, 40 of whom were asthmatics and 51 suffering from rhinitis. There is a test which is called a RAST test and this is short for radio allergosorbent test. This test measures the level of IgE antibodies in the blood to specific substances. A RAST-Candida albicans was done in 64 cases. Results were positive in 52 patients, and in 46 of these there was a correlation between the RAST and the provocation test. Hyposensitization (desensitization) treatment was given to 92 patients. After two years of treatment a good to excellent response could be observed in almost 60 per cent of the treated cases. A rough estimation of the incidence of immediate bronchial and nasal hypersensitivity among patients with chronic asthma and rhinitis to the three yeasts gave the approximate figure of 8–10 per cent. Again, this study would suggest that hypersensitivity to this organism, rather than infection, is the key mechanism involved in producing the effect.

In 1994, in a study by the University of Virginia, there was a favourable response in a group of asthmatic patients to anti-fungal therapy. In a controlled study, 10 trichophyton-allergic asthma patients were randomized to receive either 22 weeks or 44 weeks of oral fluconazole (Diflucan) 100 mg daily. After 10 months of the study, specific bronchial reactivity to Trichophyton tonsurans had shown a definite decrease in nine out of the 10 patients tested. No adverse reactions to the drugs were noted.[8] A second abstract published in the same issue of the *Journal of Allergy and Clinical Immunology*[9] came from Belgian researchers, who described the response of some of their asthmatic patients to a systemic azol anti-fungal drug. Ten corticosteroid-dependent asthmatic patients, aged 13–62, without evidence of fungal infection, entered a double-blind placebo-controlled study. The observers found that four out of the five treated patients improved after two weeks, while four of the five placebo group did not improve. This is particularly significant, as these asthmatic patients showed no evidence of fungal infection.

The Candida Phenomenon

Like most of life, the whole Candida problem centres around balance. On one side of the equation is Candida albicans, on the other side is the resistance of the host. Although Candida has in the past been regarded as an innocent commensal of the digestive tract, mycology (the study of moulds and fungi) has demonstrated that Candida albicans is very complex. It releases at least 79 known chemical substances, against which the human body creates an identifiable antibody. There are in fact 81 strains of Candida albicans, and each strain can produce 35 separate antigens. Varying strains can colonize the gut of the same person at different times in his or her life. A healthy individual has these organisms present only in small quantities in the gastro-intestinal tract, and in such people no harm results.

Candida albicans is an opportunistic organism. It will grow spectacularly when an individual's resistance is lowered or when it is particularly encouraged by factors occurring in someone's lifestyle. Resistance can be lowered by an infection, nutritional deficiencies, or some debilitating agent in the environment. Factors in our modern lifestyle that are important are high consumption of antibiotics, the contraceptive pill, and cortisone. High sugar and yeast consumption are very important, especially the sugar consumption.

When conditions are ripe for Candida proliferation, it tends to change in shape from its normal yeast-like form to a mycelial fungal form. Candida albicans is thus called a dimorphic organism because it can exist in two separate shapes. The yeast-like form is thought to be non-invasive and probably harmless. The fungal form, however, has long root-like mycelia, which can penetrate the mucous membrane lining of the intestines. This penetration of the mucosal lining can lead to 'leaky' mucous membranes (this can be seen with an electron microscope). Such a leaky mucosa is of enormous importance as it can allow incompletely digested dietary proteins, etc. to come into direct contact with the immune system. The outposts of the immune system lie underneath the mucous membranes and they are designed to deal with food which has been broken down by digestive enzymes and which is thus of low molecular weight. The contact between the immune system and these unbroken-down foodstuffs is an obvious mechanism for the production of food allergy or sensitivity. Hence, patients who have a chronic overgrowth of Candida albicans and a high percentage of the mycelial form frequently show a wide variety of food and environmental allergies.

Patients with multiple food and chemical sensitivities may become that way because antibodies were formed to the antigenic proteins in foods, pollens and even, importantly, to their own intestinal flora. In addition to causing a leaky mucosa it has now been convincingly demonstrated that Candida produces a specific toxin called Candida toxin which seems to weaken the immune system in general and make it less able to cope with other allergy problems. In particular, Candida toxin suppresses the T-lymphocytes in our immune defence systems, and as these cells are referred to as the 'generals' of that system, the immune system tends to perform in a rather disorganized manner. It is thought that when neutralization therapy for food and inhalant allergies (*see Chapters 12–14*) is not working well, it is usually because of a poorly functioning immune system and is accompanied by depressed levels of T-lymphocytes. Many failures of neutralization become successes after Candida treatment.

Candida treatment is thought to lead to a reduction in gut permeability, and it is very noticeable clinically that further food sensitivities seem much less likely to occur. In difficult, complex, refractory-type patients, Candida treatment tends to stabilize them and make them easier to treat. Minor food sensitivities often disappear, and neutralization levels (*see Chapter 12*) remain much more stable.

Diagnosis

The diagnosis that chronic intestinal candidasis is important in a specific patient is based on the whole clinical picture, established by taking a history from the patient. There are currently in the US various experimental blood tests described in detail in the book *The Yeast Syndrome* by Dr. J. P. Trowbridge and Morton Walker (Bantam Books). They include a Candida Antigen Profile, the Candi-sphere Serodiagnostic Analysis, and the Candida albicans Antibody Titer Test. These tests are undergoing long-term evaluation at the moment and may be found to be very helpful.

In asthma sufferers, the starting point for the diagnosis is often negative skin tests for inhalants and a poor response to an elimination diet, combined with a highish score on the Candida questionnaire. (In Chapter 10 you will find an extensive questionnaire, part of which relates to the Candida hypersensitivity problem.) This questionnaire is singly the most important tool in diagnosing this problem. After the questionnaire, the skin test for Candida has some distinct value, but ultimately a therapeutic trial, a technique well known and respected in other areas of medicine, is the ultimate test.

The classic clinical picture consists of the existence of: (a) predisposing factors; and (b) clinical symptoms.

Factors which predispose to chronic intestinal candidiasis are:

- Recurrent or prolonged treatment with antibiotics. All physicians know that antibiotics stir up intestinal candidiasis, but what they are not so universally aware of is the long-term adverse effects that can thereby accrue. The worst antibiotics in this respect are the broad-spectrum antibiotics such as tetracycline. These antibiotics kill a lot of the more innocent micro-organisms in the digestive tract and thereby encourage Candida albicans. The worst single example of this is the practice of treating teenage acne with courses of tetracycline, often extending over several years. I have seen many patients who have had severe problems after such treatment.

- Prolonged use of the contraceptive pill. Quite how the pill produces this effect is not well understood, but there is no doubt that it does. The original thought was that the pill stirred up candidiasis because it was a steroid, and steroids have a general depressive effect on the immune system. One of the immune system's roles is keeping gut microbes in the gut where they belong, rather than in the body's tissues, but the steroids in the pill are female sex hormones and they do not act in quite the same way as other corticosteroids. However, there does seem to be a relationship between the level of the female sex hormones oestrogen and progesterone and the ease with which Candida affects the body. Thus, there seems to be a specific interaction between the sex hormones and Candida, and this may explain why candidiasis is much more common in women generally, as well as showing how the pill influences candidiasis.

- Prolonged treatment with cortisone or cortisone-derived drugs for any particular reason.
- Multiple pregnancies.
- An environment containing a high proportion of mould. There is a fascinating interaction between environmental moulds and Candida albicans. People with severe candidiasis frequently are particularly bad in the mould season of the year, which in the UK is August, September and early October. These individuals tend to be particularly bad on damp, humid days in August and September when the mould count is clearly high. They will frequently be improved dramatically by desensitization to moulds, in addition to their Candida treatment. If a sufferer lives in a damp house with a lot of mould on the walls in the bathroom and in the kitchen, steps should be taken to eradicate these moulds as far as possible. Various techniques have been described in relation to this, described in Chapter 5.
- A history of high consumption of sugar in the past. A lot of Candida sufferers crave sugar in any form, and in fact it is one of the diagnostic features of the condition. Frequently the craving amounts to a total addiction.
- Ingestion of large quantities of yeast products.

It will be noticed that all these predisposing factors, with the exception of environmental moulds and pregnancies, are items which have steadily increased with advancing 'civilization'.

Yeast started to be used by human beings about 8,000 years ago, but only in a small way. Nowadays yeast products occur prolifically in our diet. Yeast is present in all leavened breads, all alcoholic beverages, most cheeses, mushrooms, and most fruit juices. The consumption of sugar, which was totally unknown in Europe prior to the 16th century, has increased spectacularly throughout this century, with the consumption of sugar per head of the population increasing by more than 30-fold since the beginning of the 20th century.

Antibiotics have been with us to some extent since 1942, but most of the broad-spectrum antibiotics did not arrive until the mid- and late 1940s. Cortisone and the contraceptive pill began to be used in the 1950s. All these items are now being used in progressively increasing quantities.

Symptoms Suggestive of Intestinal Candidiasis

Candida can lead to an enormous range of symptom manifestations. The most common and characteristic are:

- bloating and gaseous distention of the abdomen
- chronic rectal irritation
- repeated or chronic thrush vaginitis
- recurrent bouts of what is frequently called cystitis when it is in fact cystourethritis (bacteriological cultures of the urine are negative and there is no direct specific evidence of Candida albicans because the infection is deep in the cells of the urethra and bladder)
- recurring depression, irritability, inability to concentrate and problems with memory
- chronic nervous indigestion-type symptoms, especially in the upper part of the digestive tract (these symptoms are often erroneously diagnosed as hiatus hernia)
- chronic constipation, sometimes alternating with diarrhoea
- recurring fungal-type rashes in different parts of the body.

Virtually nobody has all of these symptoms and, of course, they can be the result of processes other than Candida. The presence of a fair number of these symptoms is highly suggestive of the problem, but what absolutely clinches the diagnosis is that these symptoms are aggravated by factors which classically aggravate thrush – in other words, they are often made worse by courses of antibiotics or large consumptions of sugar and yeast.

Treatment

The treatment of chronic intestinal candidiasis is usually a fairly prolonged business and at times can be quite difficult. Practitioners currently use one of the following five methods: (1) nystatin plus diet; (2) caprylic acid plus diet; (3) Diflucan or Sporanox plus diet; (4) amphotericin-B plus diet; and (5) Lactobacillus acidophilus plus diet. Diet is extremely important in the treatment of candidiasis, probably half the total treatment. Intestinal thrush is quite resistant to treatment and so we have to starve the thrush out by depriving it of what it thrives on, and attack it with various medications. The absolutely ideal diet to combat thrush would contain no carbohydrates at all, but this would be dangerous to the general health of the individual. The Anti-Candida diet, therefore, represents a reasonable compromise between the nutritional needs of the individual and the speed with which the ultimate result needs to be attained. Of course, the degree of restriction also depends to some extent on the severity of the individual's Candida problem.

All physicians who have treated this problem are agreed that sugar is the most important single item to be avoided. This food is the most easily available source of nutrition for Candida, which proliferates rapidly when it can obtain sugar. All sugars should be restricted and this includes cane sugar, beet sugar, glucose, powdered fructose, honey, and maple syrup. I allow my patients to eat some fruits (which, of course, contain fructose), but I instruct them to eat only those that contain the least fructose.

Having experimented with varying degrees of restriction, I have now settled on the following initial diet, which although fairly restrictive, usually leads to an obvious improvement if combined with an effective anti-fungal medication in about two to three months. If the diet is less restrictive, improvement usually takes longer, and if that happens one might run into a 'credibility gap'.

Therefore, for most people I recommend the following diet for approximately two months, although they may let up on it a bit if obvious improvement occurs with a few weeks.

Anti-Candida Diet

Phase I

To be followed for at least eight weeks.
The following foods *only*:

1. all vegetables
2. potatoes, potato flour, rice, rice pasta (Pastariso), organic rice puffs (Kallo), rice cakes, rice flour, cornflour (corn starch)
3. various oils, including sunflower oil, tahini, sesame oil, olive oil, linseed oil, safflower oil and butter
4. all meats
5. all salt water and freshwater fish. All shellfish, including prawns, crab, winkles, whelks, mussels, etc.
6. a limited number of fruits – avocado, rhubarb, lemon, lime, guava and melon
7. cow's milk - in small quantities, goat's milk, sheep's milk and non-fermented cheese such as Edam, Gouda, soft cream cheese and cottage cheese
8. all soya products
9. tea, China tea, herbal teas of all sorts, carrot juice, tomato juice and water
10. all herbs and spices.

After there has been considerable improvement, which should occur within 8–10 weeks, the diet can be expanded into the Phase II Anti-Candida Diet, which can include:

Phase II

1. fresh ground coffee
2. all grains, including wheat, oats, barley, rye wheat pasta, soda bread
3. medium sugar-containing fruits such as satsuma, strawberry, apple, cherry, blackberry, gooseberry, peach, pineapple, pomegranate
4. nuts – consumed in small quantities
5. pulses.

Improvement should continue on this expanded diet, which can then after a further couple of months be expanded in most cases into Phase III, which returns the diet to almost normal, with the notable exception of the sugar products.

Phase III

It may now be possible to introduce yeast-related foods, but it is wise to check for any yeast sensitivity at this point. This can be done by consuming three brewer's yeast tablets and noting any adverse response over the next 24/48 hours.

If there is no such response, then wholemeal bread, all cheeses, vinegar, mushrooms and alcoholic beverages low in sugar can be consumed – these would include dry wines, vodka, whisky, gin but would exclude fortified wines, liquers, sweet wines etc.

All other fruits can now be introduced; hence the only food being avoided at this stage is sugar.

When the patient is well, sugar is allowed at times in small quantities, but most patients who suffer from this problem are advised never to return to major sugar consumption. Patients almost invariably report that if they consume a lot of sugar in one form or another, they get a recurrence of symptoms. Thus, sauces, cakes, biscuits, sorbets, ice-creams, cola and other soft drinks, for most people, should be limited almost indefinitely.

Nystatin

The most effective medication to reduce the colonies of Candida albicans is nystatin. Nystatin has been used by doctors for over 30 years and has an enviable safety record. This safety record is partly because, except at very high dosage, Nystatin is not absorbed at all from the alimentary canal. In other words, it does not reach the bloodstream, but remains inside the digestive tract, where it does all its work, killing the yeast germs situated therein. An illustration of the safety of this medication comes from the cancer institutes in the US, where some children were found to be suffering from virulent intestinal candidiasis as a result of the cytotoxic drugs that they had been given. Doses of 100 tablets a day or more of nystatin were used to treat these conditions and were found to be perfectly well tolerated. Nystatin is arguably the safest medication in the British Pharmacopoeia.

Most of the doctors I know use pure nystatin powder rather than nystatin tablets, which are obtainable at the chemist. I use pure nystatin powder because it is much cheaper than the tablets which, when the full dosage is obtained, can be prohibitively expensive; the Candida organisms colonize the whole digestive tract from the mouth to the rectum and, of course, tablets which are swallowed will not treat the organisms in the mouth or the oesophagus; the tablets contain food colourings and other chemicals and filling agents, such as cornflour – these can contribute to allergy problems or compromise an elimination diet; worst of all, the tablets are sugar-coated, which somewhat defeats a sugar-free diet.

The nystatin powder must be stored in a refrigerator, but not in the freezer compartment. The most usual regimen is to start taking nystatin at a dosage of half a level teaspoon per day. The teaspoon should be a 5-ml plastic measuring teaspoon. The half-teaspoon dosage is placed into any cold drink that does not contain sugar or yeast, and stirred well until it dissolves. This total daily dose of half a teaspoon is taken in four equal doses and spread at roughly equal intervals throughout the day. Ideally the powder should be taken an hour or two before food is ingested. After a week, if there are no problems, the dosage is increased to three-quarters of a teaspoon. In most cases, the dose is thereafter increased by one-quarter of a teaspoon every week until a total dosage of 2½ teaspoons a day is attained.

At my clinic in Banstead, Surrey, we are able to supply our patients with pure nystatin powder in gelatine capsules. We have an arrangement with a pharmaceutical capsuling company who produce the pure nystatin capsules for us. The capsuling process is quite expensive and the cost of the capsules works out over twice as expensive as the pure powder. As the powder is fiddly to prepare each day and has a poor taste, many of my patients tell me that the extra expense is worth every penny. Each capsule contains a quarter teaspoon of nystatin powder, so the starting dose is two capsules a day, rising to a top dosage of 10 capsules a day.

The Herxheimer Response (Die-off Reaction)

This is the name given to certain problems that can occur with some people as the dose of nystatin is increased. The problems do not occur only with nystatin but can occur with any medication that is effectively killing Candida organisms. The more effective the medication, the more likely is the problem to occur.

In some individuals, as the dosage of nystatin is increased they may, at a certain dosage level, notice a sudden increase in the severity of the very symptoms they are treating. Sometimes, in addition, headache, fatigue, depression and flu-like symptoms may also make an appearance. These symptoms are almost certainly caused by a sudden large increase in the production of Candida toxin. Nystatin kills Candida germs quite brutally, and in laboratory tests it can be shown that the cell wall of Candida albicans disintegrates, releasing the Candida toxin held within that cell wall. Therefore, if large quantities of Candida are killed there is a large release of Candida toxin in the digestive tract. Candida toxin is absorbed from the digestive tract into the bloodstream and can lead to symptoms in any part of the body.

When the dosage of nystatin is lowered by about half a teaspoon the symptoms will usually die away in three or four days. After another week of two of nystatin treatment at the slightly reduced dosage the individual will then usually be able to tolerate the dosage of nystatin which previously produced the Herxheimer response, as more of the Candida germs have now been eliminated.

This response is named after Dr. Herxheimer, who in the early part of the 20th century described a similar response when patients were being successfully treated for syphilis. In the cases he observed, the syphilitic lesions could be shown to regress but the patient often started to experience joint pains and fever because of the toxin released by the dead spirochaetes (syphilis germs).

Anyone experiencing this type of response can be virtually certain that he or she has a Candida problem, as people without the Candida problem have no trouble at all in taking any reasonable dose of nystatin. I have always thought that obvious Herxheimer responses are probably the single most certain positive diagnostic indicator of the Candida problem.

There are some people, it must be said, who have a great deal of trouble getting on at all with nystatin. These are usually those who look pale and ill, with multiple food and chemical sensitivities. They can have decidedly adverse reactions to even micro-doses of nystatin and usually need, at least initially, to be treated with small doses of something like caprylic acid or Lactobacillus acidophilus. There are a few people who will even have Herxheimer reactions to these milder regimes, and who need to be treated with diet only, for a month or two, before any other type of active treatment can be initiated.

Various manoeuvres can be tried in this type of person to get through the early stages of effective anti-Candida treatment.

1. Candida neutralization. The technique entails finding a neutralizing level of Candida albicans in the same way as other neutralization therapy (*see Chapter 12*). The patient then takes daily subcutaneous injections of Candida extract which can produce a considerable immediate symptom improvement, and seem to counteract the Herxheimer reaction. In some patients, however, the neutralizing level is rather unstable and has to be adjusted frequently.
2. Temporarily (for about 10–14 days) eliminate all carbohydrate from the diet, while rapidly increased doses of nystatin are taken, and in these circumstances the doses can be well tolerated.
3. Colonic wash-outs to eliminate excess Candida from the colonic area, where they are usually at their most prolific.

Amphotericin-B

This is an anti-fungal antibiotic which has a mode of action identical to that of nystatin. Like nystatin, it is not absorbed from the gut except in extremely high dosage. Data from many sources indicate that this drug is a safe alternative to nystatin and can be valuable: (a) to those who do not tolerate nystatin; (b) to those having a poor clinical response to nystatin; or (c) to those who symptomatically relapse while taking nystatin, despite an initial apparent improvement.

Amphotericin-B is retained in the UK under the trade name of Fungilin in 100-mg tablets. I usually try to work up to the maximum dosage suggested by the makers, which is two 100-mg tablets four times a day.

In hospital practice amphotericin-B is sometimes given by intravenous injection. Giving it this way is very effective in treating Candida in deeper tissues but is, however, decidedly dangerous as there is a risk of kidney damage. I would only advocate the tablet form of the medication, which is almost totally safe.

Diflucan (chemical name: fluconazole)

This is a potent systemic anti-fungal drug. In contrast to nystatin and amphotericin-B, this is absorbed from the gut and does get into the bloodstream and from there to all parts of the body, including the lungs. Considering that it is distributed throughout the body, it is a remarkably safe drug; the only queries concerning its safety relate to patients who are severely ill already, with conditions such as AIDS and cancer. Except in such patients, there is no suggestion of side-effects in the liver, kidney or other organs, and it has now totally replaced Nizoral (chemical name: ketoconazole) in my affections. Occasionally, I did use Nizoral in the past when it looked as if a systemic anti-fungicide would be invaluable, but one had to monitor liver function frequently (in particular by blood test) as there was a well-documented risk (1 in 10,000) of severe hepatitis with this drug.

There are certainly patients who seem to need a systemic anti-fungicide over and above the intra-lumenal anti-fungals, such as nystatin and amphotericin-B. I see the role of nystatin and amphotericin-B being to reduce the gut reservoir and hence the source of the infection, and that of Diflucan as being to finish off the job by eradicating problems in the tissues once the gut reservoir is low. Certainly, clinically we have often seen major further improvement with Diflucan over and above that which we have obtained with nystatin.

I give Diflucan in dosage of one 50-mg capsule a day for six weeks at the most. Diflucan has only been on the market for a few years and its safety for longer courses has not been established. Professor Sydney Baker of the Gesell Institute in the US has reported using the 200-mg capsule over the same timespan with improved results in some patients. The major 'side-effect' of this medication, however, is its price. At the time of writing it is over £30 a week retail for a course of the 50-mg tablets – over £180 for the full six weeks. You can imagine what the 200-mg capsules would cost.

Sporanox (chemical name: itraconazole)

This comes in a 100-mg capsule and is a similar drug to Diflucan in that it is absorbed from the gut and distributed throughout the system. Like Diflucan, no serious side-effects have been reported, but I have not seen quite such good results with Sporanox in relation to asthma as I have with Diflucan. Maybe this has been because of luck, or possibly because in the case of Sporanox most of the drug becomes concentrated in the skin, which makes it peculiarly satisfactory for dealing with skin problems relating to Candida. Sporanox is rather less expensive than Diflucan.

My Philosophy on Drug Usage

Some patients reading my earlier book on this subject have expressed surprise at my advocacy of these powerful drugs, so I think I should clarify my position at this point.

• I am against using drugs that exist purely to suppress symptoms without attacking the cause of those symptoms. Hence, I dislike the use of anti-wheezing drugs, painkillers, steroids, tranquillizers and so forth. I agree with the 19th-century physician Constantine Hering, who used to teach his students that the suppression of acute symptoms tends to cause chronic symptoms. I accept, however, that there are times when the use of drugs in desperate circumstances may be justified.

• I am all for the use of drugs which get at the cause of illnesses, when this is possible. If I should contract meningococcal meningitis I will be taking penicillin as fast as I can lay my hands on it. Without it I would be dead in 24 hours, with it I wouldn't. If I get tuberculosis I will be the first in the queue for Streptomycin and other potent anti-tuberculosis drugs. Most severe Candida-type problems would not get better within a reasonable timespan, in my experience, without potent antifungals. They get at the cause of the problem and they are wonderfully safe.

Caprylic Acid

This anti-fungal medication is a short-chain fatty acid, originally discovered over 30 years ago by Dr. Irene Neuhauser of the University of Illinois. The huge upsurge in interest in candidiasis has prompted various companies to dig up old research on anti-fungal substances, and this particular medication has proved to be very useful. Caprylic acid is now retailed under different names, but my current favourite is Mycopryl 400 (Biocare) which seems to work especially well because it becomes uniformally dispersed on the gut wall along the entire length of the intestine. The ultimate therapeutic dose is three capsules of Mycopryl 400 three times daily, with meals, but as with the other antifungals the dose has to be increased gradually, probably from three capsules a day slowly to nine over a period of about three weeks. If the capsules are taken just before meals this maximizes the anti-fungal effect and minimizes the belching which sometimes occurs after ingesting the capsules.

As Caprylic acid is extremely safe it is retailed as a food supplement and hence it can be bought over the counter at healthfood shops and is often advocated by naturopaths, chiropractors, etc., unlike nystatin, amphotericin-B, Diflucan and Sporanox, which are only available on a doctor's prescription. The manufacturers of Mycopryl 400 suggest that its value may be enhanced if a high-yield Lactobacillus acidophilus preparation is given at the same time. As with any other product that kills Candida effectively, it can lead to the Herxheimer or die-off reaction, and as with the other medications, the problem can usually be solved by temporarily reducing the dosage and then gradually increasing it again after more of the Candida cells have been eradicated. It is noticeable that the Herxheimer reactions with this product tend to be mild and infrequent.

Lactobacillus Acidophilus

This is a non-chemical approach to Candida. It is a micro-organism which normally resides in the digestive tract of all people. On average, an adult will have approximately 2½ pounds of various micro-organisms present in the lower small intestine and colon. Lactobacillus acidophilus figures prominently in this population of micro-organisms and is wholly beneficial. There are over 200 known strains of Lactobacillus acidophilus. My current preference in regard to acidophilus products is Bio-Acidophilus (Biocare), which contains the human strain of Lactobacillus acidophilus, as opposed to the cow (bovine) strain. The human strain is also in the Lamberts product called Super Acidophilus Plus. It is considered that the human strain will probably survive much better within the human gut than the bovine strain. This is because the conditions of high acidity and high pancreatic enzymes present in the human gut are quite different from those found in the cow's gut, and the human strain of the Lactobacillus acidophilus will survive much better for these reasons.

Lactobacillus acidophilus exerts its beneficial influence by actively competing for space on the mucous membranes of the digestive tract with colonies of Candida albicans. It is also thought to have a specific antagonistic effect on the Candida albicans. In general I find

Lactobacillus acidophilus works far more slowly and less dramatically than nystatin or amphotericin-B. Its main use, therefore, is in instances when the more potent drugs cannot be tolerated. It also aids beneficial recolonization of the gut with beneficial bacteria after Candida has been largely eliminated.

Oleic Acid and Biotin

Another couple of products which are non-chemical and helpful in combating candidiasis are oleic acid and biotin. Oleic acid is found in cold-pressed olive oil and linseed oil. It acts by inhibiting the fungal form of Candida albicans and encouraging the yeast form. It is normally taken, for example, as cold-pressed olive oil in a dosage of two teaspoons three times a day.

It has been discovered that the conversion from the yeast form of Candida albicans to the mycelial form is partly dependent upon a deficiency of biotin. It is thought that biotin, when given orally, can prevent the conversion of Candida to its mycelial form. It is usually taken in a dosage of 500 mcg twice daily.

Garlic

This foodstuff has been used for medicinal purposes for centuries. Many scientific papers have now been published on the effects of garlic on strains of Candida albicans. One study, for example, showed that 24 out of 26 strains of Candida albicans were sensitive to aqueous dilutions of garlic extract. No large-scale controlled clinical trials of garlic have ever been conducted or are likely to be. The cost of such trials is huge and if they strongly support the efficacy of garlic as an anti-fungal agent, who is going to make any substantial money out of retailing a substance that cannot be patented? This is a dreadful but mostly true comment on some factors that influence medical progress.

Eminent physicians who have studied garlic state that it is a highly effective anti-fungal agent. Amounts small enough on your breath not to create a social problem will have beneficial effects. The major chemical constituent of whole garlic which gives it its therapeutic effectiveness is allicin, which is also responsible for garlic's odour. Removing the allicin to remove the odour will also remove the anti-fungal effect. Garlic powder and whole garlic cloves are undoubtedly effective, but there is a distinct question mark in my mind as to the effectiveness of the odourless preparations.

There is currently a great deal of discussion as to the various merits and demerits of the anti-fungal substances I have just described. In general, treatment of Candida has fallen into two distinct camps. On one side are the allopathic physicians who are legally entitled to prescribe anti-fungal medications such as nystatin and amphotericin-B. These physicians also employ diets similar to the one described earlier in this chapter. Another route is followed by alternative health therapists, such as chiropractors and naturopaths, who are legally unable to prescribe these drugs. They rely on caprylic acid, Lactobacillus acidophilus, garlic, oleic acid and biotin. In common with other allopathic physicians, I make quite a lot of use of the more natural anti-fungal medications in patients who are particularly sensitive to the Herxheimer-type response.

Neutralization Therapy for Candidiasis

Another treatment used by many allergists treating this problem is vaccination using extracts of Candida albicans. I use Candida albicans extract in varying strengths, in the same way as I use food or inhalant extracts to neutralize patients to foods or inhalants, as described in Chapters 12 and 13. Neutralizing doses of Candida albicans can be spectacularly effective in helping the patient, especially in the short term. The response is sometimes so dramatic that it totally convinces the patient that the problems are related to Candida albicans.

The disadvantage of this treatment is that the neutralizing level of Candida albicans has an awkward habit of changing rather rapidly, necessitating retesting at frequent intervals. Sometimes desensitization with TCE, which is a mixture of trichophyton, Candida albicans and epidermophyton, can be even more successful.

Thus, in summary, Candida albicans, trichophyton and epidermophyton are a quite significant cause of approximately 8–10 per cent of all asthma. When one considers that several million people suffer from this condition, 10 per cent represents an awful lot of people.

The Role of Magnesium and Other Nutrients

There is overwhelming evidence that some nutrients play a role in the development and maintenance of asthma. The four which have been identified are:

1. The mineral magnesium
2. Vitamin B_{12}
3. Vitamin B_6
4. Vitamin C.

Magnesium

There are many minerals which are essential to human health. The importance of iron and calcium is generally recognized, but most people outside the realm of nutritional medicine have little knowledge of the vital role of minerals such as zinc, magnesium, chromium, manganese, selenium and molybdenum. There are countless clinical papers exploring the role of these minerals in human health and yet most physicians are taught none of this during their medical education.

Deficiencies of magnesium and other minerals have increased markedly since the Second World War, and this situation has been allowed to continue as a result of the lack of interest in this area by the medical profession as a whole. Amongst the most important reasons why mineral deficiencies are developing are:

- Poor soils and commercial growing practices. Commercially grown vegetables are fertilized with the minerals that make them look good, but not necessarily good nutrition-wise. Commercially grown produce often has less than 75 per cent of the nutritional content that is found in organically-grown produce.

- Chronic exposure to chemicals depletes our nutrient pool as we struggle to detoxify them (*see Chapter* 7).
- Acid rain bleaches minerals out of soils.
- Cooking destroys many vitamins, and a lot of minerals are lost to the water.
- Chronic disease and age decrease the absorption of minerals and other nutrients.
- Food processing removes a large percentage of minerals and vitamins from food.

A recent US Government survey[1] states that the average American consumes less than 40 per cent of the recommended daily allowance of magnesium. Dr. Mildred Seelig, one of the leading authorities in the US on the subject of magnesium, suggests that 80–90 per cent of the American population is notably magnesium-deficient.

Returning to the role of minerals in asthma, there is no strong evidence that any mineral, other than magnesium, plays a major role. However, if we think back to the chapter on chemical sensitivity it will be recalled that molybdenum, zinc and selenium are all involved in the detoxification of chemicals which, of course, is important in patients who react adversely to chemicals.

Therefore, when it comes to considering asthma, the mineral that stands out head and shoulders above all others is magnesium. Its role in the causation of this condition has been established and studied from all sorts of angles, and the progressive reduction in the content of magnesium in farming soils is, in my opinion, one of the major contributing causes of the asthma epidemic sweeping many countries of the world, especially since the 1950s.

How then, precisely, does magnesium influence asthma? The evidence is that it works in two ways, which are probably complementary to each other.

1. *Broncho-spasm relaxation*. Magnesium is essential for both voluntary muscle (striated) and involuntary (smooth) muscle relaxation. Calcium, in contrast, is necessary for the contraction. Voluntary muscles are those which we are aware of and which enable us to move and lift. Smooth or involuntary muscles are present in many areas of the body, such as the gut, but of especial interest in this context are the bronchial tubes. Thus, if the bronchial tubes go into spasm as a result of an allergic reaction, for example to dust mite, they will find

it harder to relax out of that spasm if inadequate magnesium is present. Intravenous magnesium has been used for years as a way of treating acute asthma, and I think that it is likely that if magnesium is so useful when the asthmatic is in dire straits, it is pretty likely that he or she would be better off having adequate levels of this mineral around before the problem started.

2. *Magnesium deficiency causes mast cell instability.* Mast cells are those cells which liberate histamine in response to an allergic reaction. Histamine then goes on to initiate the spasm of the bronchial tubes. This phenomenon was shown to occur in rats in experiments performed at Brigham Young University in Utah.[2] This study concluded that both the blood and urinary histamine levels of immunized severely magnesium-deficient rats were significantly higher than those of all the other groups throughout the study, particularly after specific antigen challenges. They also stated that there was a synergism of antigen challenge and severe magnesium deficiency on blood and urinary histamine levels. The results suggest that severe magnesium deficiency can aggravate diseases which are caused by abnormal histamine release, such as asthma.

This discovery was then tested in human beings at the University of Turin in a paper entitled 'Reduction of Histamine Induced Bronchoconstriction by Magnesium in Asthmatic Subjects'.[3] The authors concluded that they had observed a significant decrease in histamine induced broncho-constriction after the inhalation of magnesium sulphate in asthmatics with mild to moderate bronchial hyper-reactivity. In August 1994 *The Lancet* published a huge study involving 2,633 adults between the ages of 18 and 70 from Nottingham in England and Boston in the US. The study was entitled 'Dietary Magnesium, Lung Function, Wheezing, and Airways Hyper-reactivity in a Random Adult Population Sample'. This major study concluded that the dietary requirement of magnesium may be as high as 420 mg per day. However, a typical diet in the UK provides an estimated average of 323 mg a day in men and 237 mg a day in women. Thus, a substantial proportion of the UK adult population is magnesium-deficient. The study found that a high magnesium intake was associated with a decrease in the relative risk of airway hyper-reactivity independent of other factors, and that the magnitude of this effect was substantial. Those patients who consumed a lot of magnesium had only half of the airway hyper-reactivity as compared with those on the lowest intake.[4] This study, because of the huge number of people involved, and because of the high status of the two institutions involved in carrying it out, would be exceedingly difficult to refute. It does, I think, show beyond all reasonable doubt that magnesium plays an extremely important role in causing asthma.

To complete the case for the role of magnesium in asthma, I should mention three other trials which point to the same conclusion.

1. 28 patients with atopic asthma were studied, both during an exacerbation and when without symptoms, and they were compared to three healthy controls. During an asthma attack, blood and red blood cell magnesium decreased. The extent of the decrease was inversely correlated with the rise in histamine level and the number of eosinophils in the blood.[5]

2. Experimental double-blind study: 38 patients suffering from acute exacerbations of moderate to severe asthma randomly received either 1.2g of magnesium sulphate or placebo, after B-antagonist therapy failed to produce any significant improvement. The group given the magnesium demonstrated an increase in peak expiratory flow rate from 225 to 297 litres per minute, as compared with 208 to 216 litres per minute in the placebo group. In addition, the number admitted to hospital versus those discharged was significantly lower for the magnesium treated group.[6]

3. Experimental double-blind study: Intravenously administered magnesium significantly improved pulmonary function of asthmatic patients. The degree of improvement was positively correlated with serum magnesium levels.[7]

The Management of Magnesium Deficiency

Thus when I see a patient with asthma, I will always want to know what the magnesium status of that particular patient is.

The Red Blood Cell Magnesium Level

This test is available in many hospital pathology laboratories. It should be emphasized that it is the red blood cell magnesium level that needs to be measured and *not* a serum magnesium level, which is almost worthless. The level of magnesium in the serum fluctuates hugely throughout the day and night and magnesium passes through the serum very quickly. As such the 'normal' levels have to be set enormously wide and make the result meaningless.

Sweat Test

A very specialized laboratory, the Biolab Medical Unit in London, offers a sweat test, the results of which correlate remarkably closely with the red blood cell magnesium level. A patch is placed on the patient's back and left *in situ* for an hour while he or she remains in the waiting room. After an hour the patch is removed and placed into an atomic absorption photo-spectrometer, which then very accurately measures the amount of magnesium in the sweat, in billionths of a gram. I have found this test remarkably valuable, and one can observe increases in the level of magnesium in the sweat after giving the patient appropriate magnesium supplements.

The Magnesium Retention (or Loading Test)

This test involves collecting a complete 24-hour urine sample. Every drop of urine that is excreted for 24 hours is collected in a jug and analysed for magnesium content by the laboratory. When this 24 hours has elapsed the patient is given an injection of 2cc. magnesium sulphate intra-muscularly and then the amount of magnesium in the next 24 hours' worth of urine is estimated. The amount of magnesium excreted in the second 24 hours is then compared with the amount excreted in the first 24 hours. If the patient is very magnesium-deficient he or she will have soaked up all this magnesium sulphate, given by injection, like a sponge, and so there will be very little increase in the second urine specimen. In contrast, if the patient has an adequate magnesium level before the injection, most of the extra magnesium will be excreted in the urine that follows that injection.

Myothermogram

This is a test which is quite fascinating and has been developed by Dr. John Howard of the Biolab Medical Unit. Two heat-measuring electrodes are placed on the biceps muscle and the patient quickly shakes a fist at the operator. A curve of response is noted on the computer screen, which in a patient with normal magnesium status will look similar to the curve shown in Figure 19.

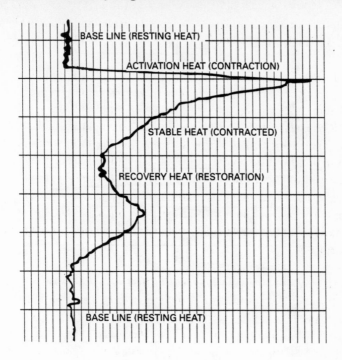

Figure 19 Myothermogram of patient with normal magnesium status

In the case of a patient with magnesium deficiency one would see a curve as shown in Figure 20.

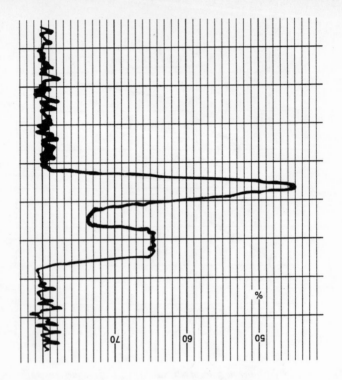

Figure 20 Patient with a magnesium deficiency

And this response becomes very exaggerated after ordinary exercise or after isometric exercise, as can be seen in Figure 21.

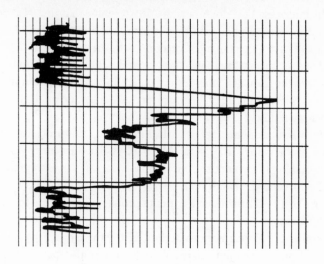

Figure 21 After mild isometric exercise

These results are extremely conclusive evidence of intracellular magnesium deficiency.

Hair Mineral Test

Magnesium deficiency also can be measured by a Hair Mineral Test, which has the advantage that one can send a sample of hair quite easily to a laboratory. I personally think it is a little less accurate than some of the above methods.

Treatment of Magnesium Deficiency

As the magnesium content even of those foods historically high in magnesium content is somewhat now unreliable, most physicians have come to the conclusion that magnesium supplements are the most satisfactory way of treating deficiency. There is a whole variety of magnesium tablets and capsules available on the market. My current favourite at the moment is the slow-release magnesium, as some of the other varieties can fairly easily give patients diarrhoea, as a result of which they lose a great deal of magnesium.

If the magnesium deficiency is considerable, magnesium sulphate 50 per cent is available in 2cc. ampules which can be given intra-muscularly into the buttocks. This does have the disadvantage that the area around the injection site can be quite tender for a few hours; occasionally the patient will have quite a marked reaction in this respect.

Perhaps the nicest way to give very high doses of magnesium is intravenously in the form of a 'magnesium push': 2cc. of magnesium sulphate is diluted with about 12cc. of intravenous quality normal saline and administered slowly over a period of about 5 minutes. The patient frequently notices some degree of flushing during this procedure, but it appears to be remarkably safe. Many physicians are nervous about giving anything intravenously, but this procedure has an extremely good safety record and the results can be truly staggering. There is certainly nothing like it to confirm that a patient's problems are related to magnesium deficiency.

A number of physicians, both in the UK and the US, are giving intravenous nutrients to patients particularly with steroid-dependent asthma or to treat acute asthmatic attacks. Magnesium is the most important constituent in these intravenous infusions, but other trace minerals, vitamins and suchlike also feature. This can be extremely effective treatment for an acute attack of asthma, and in that one is replacing fundamental deficiencies, it seems to be a much better idea than nebulizers, etc. I think there will probably be a big future in giving high-dosage intravenous drip infusions to the more severely affected asthmatics to complement all the other treatment modalities described in this book. So far, we do not have enough practical experience of this to make any claims on behalf of this approach. However, I do know a number of American physicians who have been using this technique for several years who are very enthusiastic about the improvement it has produced in many of their patients.

Vitamin B$_{12}$

Jonathan V. Wright M.D., one of the most respected and innovative nutritional physicians in the US, is responsible for the concept that vitamin B$_{12}$ is important in asthma. In a paper published in 1988[8] he reported that vitamin B$_{12}$ had been a major tool in the elimination or amelioration of wheezing, of whatever cause. In other words, this vitamin was effective in treating asthma, whether it had been labelled allergic, intrinsic or just exercise-induced asthma.

Actually, the whole story began back in 1931 with the observations of Dr. George Bray of the Asthma Clinic at the Hospital for Sick Children in Great Ormond Street, London. He published his findings under the title of 'The Hypochlorhydria of Asthma in Childhood' in the *Quarterly Journal of Medicine*.[9] In this particular study, Dr. Bray found that 160 out of 200 asthmatic children were hypochlorhydric, many of them severely. Hypochlorhydria is a deficiency of the hydrochloric acid excreted by the parietal cells in the stomach, which provide the necessary acid level to prevent bacterial growth and to help with protein digestion. While talking of these parietal cells, it should be mentioned that they also excrete 'intrinsic factor', which attaches to vitamin B_{12} and is necessary for the absorption of this vitamin in the small intestine. It has been known for many years that people with low gastric acid do not assimilate vitamin B_{12} as well as people with normal amounts of this acid. The available evidence indicates that vitamin B_{12} mal-absorption is due partly to the deficiency of intrinsic factor and partly the lack of hydrochloric acid. One might have thought that giving vitamin B_{12} by tablets would overcome this problem, but perhaps the absorption is so poor in these circumstances that even high doses by mouth seem unable to do the job.

Looking at the various studies of vitamin B_{12} given by injection to asthmatic patients, it is obvious that the dosage of this vitamin is extremely important. In 1951, for example, Simon[10] reported 20 adults with intractable asthma, all given 1,000 mcg of intramuscular vitamin B_{12} once weekly, for four weeks. Eighteen of these 20 noted improvement, but in none of them was there elimination of the problem. Two of the 20 reported no change.

In contrast, work done in Italy by Caruselli *et al*[11] abstracted in the *Journal of the American Medical Association* showed much higher doses were very effective. Thirty mg (not mcg) of vitamin B_{12} were given intravenously to 12 adult asthmatics daily for 15 to 20 days. Ten of the 12 were reported to have completely relieved their wheezing. Of these 10, one had a recurrence after three months and another after eight months. Repeat treatment was successful for both. In 1957 Crockett reported work involving 85 individuals at all ages up to 60. These were given much lower doses of 1,000 mcg of vitamin B_{12} at weekly intervals, and then later in intervals of up to four weeks. Crockett reported his results as shown in the table below.

Age	Number	'Moderate' or 'Marked' Improvement	Percent Improved
0–10	6	5	83%
10–20	19	14	74%
20–30	15	10	67%
30–40	25	13	52%
40–50	13	5	38%
50–60	7	1	14%

All the researchers in this field agree that treatment with young people is much more successful than with older ones, and that dosage is clearly extremely important.

Dr. Jonathan Wright's current treatment protocol starts with intramuscular vitamin B_{12} daily for 30 days, then 3 times weekly for 2 weeks, 2 times weekly for 2 weeks, then once weekly with adjustments upwards or downwards according to response. He gives 1 cc. on each occasion to children between the ages of 1 and 3, 2 cc. for ages 3 to 10, and for all ages over 11, 3 cc. on each occasion. With this regime he reported that only one child out of one hundred did not improve at all, and approximately 60 per cent of those under the age of 10 had stopped asthma entirely, and none of this group was steroid-dependent. Wright also reported that 20 to 30 per cent had partial but sustantial relief and only 10 per cent experienced poor results. Steroid-dependency was an adverse factor in the success rate in these children.

Why such high doses of vitamin B_{12} are necessary is far from clear. The reason for giving them is purely because of the observation that these are the doses that produce the dramatic results. The actual mechanism of how vitamin B_{12} is so effective is unknown, but of course medicine is replete with examples of very successful treatments being observed to work for many years prior to an adequate explanation of why they do.

Vitamin B_{12} may eliminate or ameliorate wheezing, but it does nothing to clear underlying allergies to either inhalants or foods, etc., which still require attention. Similarly, it does not improve the gastric acid situation, which must be treated independently.

Gastric Re-acidification

Dr. George Bray, who made the original observations at Great Ormond Street Hospital regarding low gastric acid,[12] found that 160 asthmatic children found to have sub-normal levels of hydrochloric acid following a test meal, received hydrochloric acid before or during meals in addition to continued exclusion of foods to which they were known to be sensitive. There was an immediate improvement in appetite, weight, sleep and asthmatic attacks, which became shorter in duration and lesser in intensity. If offending food allergens could be identified and removed, there was an immediate freedom from asthma. However, if this wasn't possible, the attacks ceased after three or more months, depending on the initial severity of the asthma.

Vitamin B_6

There has not been a lot of work published concerning the roles of the B vitamins in asthma, other than B_{12}. In the case of vitamin B_3 (nicotinamide or niacinamide), the results of treatment have been rather equivocal. Some studies have shown some benefit and others have not. Hence, I will not bore the reader with a detailed recital of these studies.

However, in the case of vitamin B_6 (pyridoxine) there have been a number of studies that seem to prove a benefit for the use of this vitamin, so I will briefly review them.

In one experimental study, published in the *Annals of Allergy*,[13] 76 asthmatic children who received vitamin B_6 (200 mg. daily) demonstrated a significant symptom improvement and a reduction in the required dosage of bronchodilators and cortisone.

In another study, seven patients and six controls[14] received 50 mg of pyridoxine twice daily. Both plasma and red blood cell Piridoxal Phosphate levels only increased significantly in the controls. However, *all* asthmatics reported a dramatic decrease in the frequency, duration and severity of asthmatic attacks. Most wheezing had ceased within a week.

These two trials are rather interesting, and it is surprising that much larger trials have not been undertaken to clinch the role of this vitamin in asthma.

Vitamin C

Most studies show a beneficial role for vitamin C in the management of asthma, although at least one study contradicts this view. The positive studies are:

1. In a huge study of 9,074 white and black adults aged 30 and over, carefully controlled for other possible confusing factors, increased vitamin C intake was associated with a 30 per cent lower incidence of wheezing and bronchitis.[15]
2. Pre-treatment of normal subjects with 500 mg vitamin C was found to prevent nitrogen dioxide exposure from producing airway hyper-reactivity to a challenge test with metha-colene.[16]
3. Broncho-constriction brought on by a metha-colene challenge in 14 mild asthmastics was inhibited by 1 g of oral vitamin C.[17]
4. Experimental double-blind study of 41 Nigerian children showed that those who received 1,000 mg of vitamin C daily for 14 weeks had fewer than one-quarter as many asthma attacks as those receiving placebo, and the attacks which did occur were significantly less severe. A few weeks after the vitamin C was discontinued, the frequency of attacks in the group that had improved reverted to the levels seen in the other group.[18]
5. In another study, 12 patients with exercise-induced wheezing randomly received vitamin C (500 mg daily) or a placebo. After only two days of pre-treatment with vitamin C there was significantly less wheezing seen five minutes after exercise compared to those patients who were on placebo.[19]

The negative study was on a relatively small group of 16 asthmatic adults. In this group the asthmatics failed to show any significant improvement in objective tests, such as forced expiratory volume, following the inhalation of histamine after 2 g of vitamin C. The response was the same as attained with placebo, suggesting that vitamin C had no bronchodilator effect and did not alter the reaction of the bronchiole to histamine in asthmatic adults.[20]

An Integrated Hypothesis

As a result of these observations, Dr. Jonathan Wright, who was mentioned earlier in this chapter, suggested that cow's milk and other food allergens may cause severe allergic gastritis (inflammation of the stomach) which then may result in hypochlorhydria, low pepsin secretion and a possible failure in the production of intrinsic factor. The low gastric acid and low pepsin may then result in incomplete digestion and the absorption of large molecules of undigested food, which would then go on to increase the number and severity of food allergies found to be present. This could be expected to impair micro-nutrient nutrition, and the failure of intrinsic factor production would lead to poor absorption of vitamin B_{12} and probable deficiencies in the utilization of this vitamin. Dr. Wright, therefore, proposed a programme of increasing vitamin B_{12}, vitamin B_6, magnesium, gastric re-acidification and food allergy management, and he reported the results of this strategy in three cases.[21] All three patients did remarkably well.

It might at this moment be apposite to discuss why the use of magnesium, vitamins B_{12} and B_6, vitamin C and suchlike is not common in standard medical practice. These nutrients are used by nutritional physicians, but in terms of numbers, compared to the rest of the medical profession they represent an extremely small fraction.

Whereas it is excusable, and to some extent understandable, for physicians not to get involved in the sorting out of food and inhalant sensitivities for which they have had absolutely no training, anyone can prescribe magnesium and other nutrients with only minimal knowledge. These nutrients are cheap and have no serious side-effects, whereas bronchodilator inhalers, steroid inhalers and the like are all associated with known dangers.

Very instructive in this respect was the paper published in *The Lancet*, which takes no pharmaceutical advertising. The paper was entitled 'Which anti-convulsant for women with eclampsia? Evidence from the collaborative eclampsius trial', (*Lancet* 34, September 23rd, 1995: 778–89). Eclampsia is an extremely serious condition which occurs as a result of toxaemia of pregnancy. In eclampsia, pregnant women can have severe fits, and a proportion of them die as a result. In the US since 1906, obstetricians have regarded the mineral magnesium as first-line therapy for this condition. In contrast, in England, in 1992, only 2 per cent of obstetricians routinely used magnesium as first-line therapy.

The study mentioned above was 30 times larger than any other study ever reported, and data was collected from 1,680 women with eclampsia.

Three treatments are available for this condition:

1. Diazepam (Valium)
2. Phenytoin
3. Magnesium sulphate.

All three treatments are given by injection for this condition.

In this study it was conclusively shown that women allocated magnesium had a 52 per cent lower risk of recurrent convulsions than those allocated Diazepam, and 67 per cent lower risk than those allocated Phenytoin. They were 26 per cent and 50 per cent less likely to die after magnesium sulphate than with, respectively, Diazepam or Phenytoin.

Women allocated magnesium showed many other advantages and their babies fared much better as well. The authors of this trial commented that, worldwide, about four million women have died of eclampsia since 1906 and a huge number of them could have been saved had magnesium been used in their management. This bias against the nutrient is typical of the attitude of a medical profession in love with pharmaceutical products promoted with glossy brochures, promotional conferences and an army of medical representatives.

Doctors are inevitably a product of their medical education, where only token acknowledgement is given regarding the value of nutrition in health. No attention is given to the potential use of nutrients as a specific intervention and no intellectual framework is provided with which to connect the theoretical awareness of nutritional biochemistry to the uses of nutrition as therapy. In truth, the average physician will be totally unaware of the contents of this chapter, and probably surprised by it.

This shortcoming is compounded by economic factors. Pharmaceutical companies are profit-orientated commercial enterprises with financial responsibilities to their shareholders and therefore cannot possibly be expected to operate to the detriment of their balance sheets. Nutritional supplements are in the public domain and are entirely non-patentable. Therefore, the profit margin on nutrients is very small, as anyone can make them, and pharmaceutical companies would be unable to obtain a reasonable return on their investment. One month's worth of bronchodilators and steroid inhalers is much more profitable than a month of magnesium and B vitamins. Consequently, nutritional supplements have become 'therapeutic orphans', and have not been and will not be marketed by pharmaceutical companies. Because funding for further medical education and research comes predominantly from these pharmaceutical companies, the emphasis is predominantly on the use of those pharmaceuticals from which they can obtain a profit, to the detriment of knowledge regarding nutritional and other 'unprofitable therapies'.

Such then is the way of the world, but the health of millions of people with asthma should not depend on such market forces. Leading figures in the medical profession should carefully evaluate just in what direction we are going. At this moment in time, it appears to be the wrong direction, but an investigation into the nutritional, environmental and allergic bases of asthma could change all of that.

10

What's Causing my Asthma?

Asthma is a multi-aetiologic problem. That is, in common with many chronic illnesses it has many causes, and the causes vary considerably between one patient and another. The first step, and a major one in sorting out an individual's problem, lies in the history. In allergy diagnosis, history taking and skin testing are the most important tools. In contrast, physical examination of the lungs gives virtually no answers when it comes to considering causation.

I have divided the main causes into five areas: (1) food allergy and intolerance; (2) biological inhalant sensitivity; (3) chemical sensitivity; (4) Candida hypersensitivity; and (5) magnesium deficiency. It may be noticed by the reader that some factors may appear in more than one section. For example, worsening of asthma in the early morning can be due to a night-time's exposure to the dust mite or withdrawal response to a food allergen.

A Questionnaire

Food Allergy and Intolerance

	Point Score
1. *Fatigue*:	
Slight	10
Moderate	20
Severe	30
2. *Obesity*:	
(Weight able to fluctuate by 4 lb or more within a day)	20
In addition:	
1 stone overweight	5
2 stone overweight	10
3 stone or more overweight	15

3. *Swelling and puffiness of face, ankles or fingers*:
   Slight swelling   10
   Moderate swelling   20
   Bad to the extent of needing to take diuretics (water pills)   30

4. *Bouts of sweating for no obvious cause*:   20
   (For example, waking up at night feeling hot and sweaty. This
   does not include menopausal sweats, unless they have been
   present for five years or more.)

5. *Bouts of your heart beating fast*:
   Very occasionally   10
   Frequently   20

6. *Any history of known food intolerance causing any symptoms*:
   One food known   10
   Several foods   20

7. *Any history of dependence, craving for, or addiction to such foods as*:
   Bread
   Sugar
   Chocolate   15
   Milk
   Coffee
   Tea

8. *Does the consumption of alcohol make your asthma worse the
   following morning?*
   Yes   30

9. *A history of any other condition known to be connected with food
   allergy, such as*:
   Migraine
   Severe headaches
   Irritable bowel syndrome
   Eczema   15
   Urticaria
   Depression
   Myalgia (aching muscles)

10. *Any history of abdominal bloating*   15

11. *Does missing a meal make your asthma worse?*   20

As can be seen, it is possible to score 250 points on this part of the questionnaire, but the highest I have seen in clinical practice would be around 190 points. Most people who prove to have a food allergy problem underlying their asthma would have a score of around 70 points. Anyone with a score higher than 90 could feel fairly confident that food allergy was at least part of the problem, unless there was truly overwhelming evidence of, for example, inhalant sensitivity.

A symptom score system like this can easily be criticized, as it is fairly subjective in some areas. For example, one person may consider his or her fatigue to be moderate, whereas another may consider the same fatigue to be severe. Some of the other questions, however, can only invite a straight 'yes' or 'no' response.

Biological Inhalant Sensitivity

In this section the scoring system appropriate in the other sections is not really helpful.

1. *Is the asthma present only in certain summer months?*
   If the answer to this is 'yes', it is almost conclusive that inhalant sensitivity is the whole cause of the problem.
2. *Symptoms present predominantly in March, April, May:*
   This indicates that tree pollens are likely to be implicated.
3. *Asthma present only, or much worse, in May, June and July:*
   This indicates that grass pollens are likely to be implicated.
4. *Asthma worse in August, September, into early October, ceasing after the first frost of the year:*
   This would suggest mould spores are likely to be implicated.
5. *Symptoms present all year round, but definitely worse in the summer:*
   This indicates that summer pollens are implicated, but the all-year-round symptomatology could be due to dust mite and mould sensitivities, food sensitivities, chemical sensitivities, etc.
6. *Asthma worse before rain, especially thunder storms:*
   A rise in humidity before rain encourages mould spore production.
7. *Asthma worse with grass cutting:*
   Both grasses and moulds are stirred up from the ground by this procedure.
8. *Asthma worse in the early hours of morning in July and August:*
   Moulds, including basidiospores, are shed in huge numbers in the right conditions.
9. *Asthma worse on turning over compost heap:*
   Compost is saturated with moulds and many spores are liberated when the compost is turned over.

10. *Asthma worse near combine harvesters or other harvesting*:
    A huge cloud of mould spores follows a combine harvester and the drivers of these machines are advised to wear masks to give them some protection.
11. *Asthma worse near feathers.*
12. *Asthma worse in dry summer*:
    Grass pollen counts are higher in these circumstances.
13. *Asthma worse in wet summer*:
    Mould counts are higher in these circumstances.
14. *Asthma worse in winter*:
    House dust and dust mite sensitivity is likely in these circumstances. Dust mites are encouraged by humidity in hermetically-sealed houses. Ducted central heating systems move dust around the house. Indoor moulds like Penicillium are more prevalent in damp basements.
15. *Asthma worse on waking in the morning*:
    Dust and dust mite sensitivity is likely.
16. *Asthma worse at night in bed*:
    Dust and dust mites are likely, as are pets if allowed into the bedroom.
17. *Asthma worse indoors*:
    Usually dust, dust mite, moulds or pets.
18. *Asthma improved or completely better on holidays abroad in hot, very dry circumstances like arid Greek islands, the Portuguese Algarve, Arizona and Tunisia*:
    Assuming the asthma sufferer is staying in rooms with no carpets, there is no appreciable dust or moulds in these circumstances. Dust mite does not exist at all. This observation is almost totally conclusive in diagnosis of inhalant sensitivity, although occasionally this can be misleading, as a patient with a cow's milk intolerance may improve in the Greek Islands where there is very little cow's milk.
19. *Asthma non-existent at high altitudes, as in ski-ing holidays*:
    No dust mite or mould in these circumstances. Observation almost certainly indicative of biological inhalant sensitivity.
20. *Asthma worse on holidays in Florida, Malaysia, Thailand, etc.*:
    The combination of heat and high humidity encourages mould growth. This observation almost diagnostic for mould sensitivity.

Many patients know long before they consult a physician or read a book like this that animals such as cats, dogs, or horses can provoke an immediate asthmatic attack on close contact.

Chemical Sensitivity

Any person noticing an asthmatic response while in contact with any of the following has at least a partial chemical sensitivity. As pointed out earlier (*see Chapter* 7), reactions to gas, oil, cigarette smoke and formaldehyde are much more important, as these pollutants are present almost continuously in many homes and, because the exposure is continuous, people do not notice an adverse response. Intermittent-type exposures, if positive, are awarded 10 points on the score, and the more pernicious and generally harmful chemicals are awarded 20 points if the patient is aware that he or she is reacting to some extent to them.

		Point Score
1.	Petrol	10
2.	Diesel	10
3.	Gas cooker and/or boiler (if installed indoors)	20
4.	Oil boiler (if installed indoors)	20
5.	Gloss paint	10
6.	Perfumes	10
7.	Cigarette or cigar smoke	20
8.	Hair sprays	10
9.	New wool carpeting	20
10.	Fabric shops	20
11.	Floor wax	10
12.	Nail polish	10
13.	Furniture polish	10
14.	Varnishes	10
15.	Deodorants	10
16.	Bleach or usage of indoor swimming pool	10
17.	Carpet shampoo	10
18.	Photocopiers	10
19.	Fresh newspapers	10
20.	Department stores	10

In this section of this questionnaire, as for that on food sensitivity, it is possible to score reasonably as shown. As with the food allergy section there is a maximum total of 250 points, but anyone who notices his or her asthma reacting to chemicals in this way has a chemical sensitivity problem. Any score in excess of 60 would almost be a firm diagnosis of the fact that chemical sensitivity is playing a role in the patient's problems.

Candida Hypersensitivity

Women are more likely to have this problem than men, probably because of their more complex hormone systems; there is a distinct link between Candida hypersensitivity and 'hormonal'-type symptomatology. This section of the questionnaire is divided into two parts: (a) predisposing factors; and (b) consequences.

Predisposing Factors

		Point Score
1.	Have you taken more than one course of antibiotics per year in the last five years?	10
	Or, alternatively, have you taken antibiotics at any time in your life for more than two months, as in treatment for acne or long-term infections?	30
2.	Do you live in a damp, mouldy house with visible mould on the walls and also, for example, around the bottom of windows?	10
3.	Do you eat a lot of sugar? Please note that soft drinks like colas etc. may have more than five teaspoons of sugar in each can. Cakes, biscuits, ice creams, sorbets, sweets, chocolate, etc. all contain a lot of sugar.	
	Moderate consumption	10
	Large consumption	15
4.	Do you consume a lot of yeasty products, such as alcohol (especially beer, wine and champagne rather than spirits), bread, cheese, mushrooms, vinegar, Marmite?	
	Moderate consumption	5
	Large consumption	10
5.	Do you suffer from diabetes?	10
6.	Steroids: Have you taken steroids, such as cortisone or prednisolone by mouth, or inhaled steroids like Becotide or steroid injections?	
	Taken for up to four weeks	5
	More than four weeks	10

Women only, for obvious reasons:

7. *Have you been pregnant?*
   Once   3
   Two or more times   5

8. *Have you taken the contraceptive pill?*
   Up to six months   5
   Up to two years   10
   More than two years   15

9. *Have you taken Hormone Replacement Therapy in tablet form?*
   For a few months   5
   Over one year   10

Thus, the maximum score in this section is 85 for men and 115 for women.

Consequences of Candida Hypersensitivity

Point Score

1. *Do you suffer from excessive wind and bloating of the abdomen, the bloating at times looking like early pregnancy?*   30

2. *Do you have indigestion and/or heartburn in the upper part of the abdomen?*   10

3. *Do you suffer from thrush, that is vaginal thrush or oral thrush in females, penile or oral thrush in males?*
   Rarely   10
   Very frequently   30

4. *Do you suffer from bowel irregularity, either:*
   (a) constipation   5
   (b) diarrhoea, or   5
   (c) constipation alternating with diarrhoea?   10

5. *Do you notice irritation around the anus?*
   Rarely   5
   Frequently   15

6. *Do you suffer from athlete's foot, ringworm, jock itch, or other long-term fungal infection of the skin or nails?*
   Occasionally   5
   Frequently   15

7. *Do you have problems with memory and concentration?*   10

8. *Do you crave sugar?*   10

9. *Are you prone to suffering with cystitis or frequency of urination with some degree of burning?*   15

   In addition, if you have urine cultures, do they usually prove negative? 5

10. *Does alcohol upset you, even if taken in small quantities?*   10

11. *Are you worse when the weather is damp?*   5

12. *Do you have a loss of sexual desire or impotence?*   10

13. *Do you suffer from psoriasis?*   10

14. *Do you have problems with poor coordination?*   5

15. *Are you sensitive to chemical odours, such as petrol fumes, diesel fumes, paint fumes, perfumes, etc.?*   10

Women Only

16. *Did the contraceptive pill upset you in some way when you first took it, for example, headache, depression or weight gain?*   10

17. *Did Hormone Replacement Therapy taken by mouth have similar adverse effects?*   10

18. *Do you feel distinctly worse premenstrually, for example with depression, tension, water retention, breast tenderness and headaches?*   10

19. *Do you suffer from endometriosis or infertility?*   5

What makes the diagnosis of Candida hypersensitivity even more likely is the observation that the consequences (the last 19 symptoms) are noticeably worse after contact with the predisposing factors, such as antibiotics, the contraceptive pill, HRT, cortisone, or high sugar, yeast or mould intake.

If the score for the predisposing factors and the consequences are added together, the maximum score for women would be 340, whereas for men it would be 280. In women, any score of less than 60 (in men less than 50) would suggest that Candida hypersensitivity is unlikely to be a factor in their illness. In both sexes scores of over 100 make the problem likely, and in anyone with a score of over 180 (women), or 140 (men), the diagnosis would be a certainty.

However, even if the Candida score is very high, it does not represent conclusive proof that this problem is the whole cause of a patient's asthma. It does indicate that the patient's general health will improve greatly if the Candida is treated, but it is possible that the asthma may still, for example, be predominantly a dust mite sensitivity. Candida, however, appears to be a very important cause of asthma in a small group of patients.

Magnesium Deficiency

Magnesium is needed for muscle relaxation, whereas calcium is needed for muscle contraction. Magnesium deficiency is responsible for a wide range of musculoskeletal disorders that are rarely diagnosed as having this cause. Some of the symptoms of magnesium deficiency centre around the neuro-psychiatric end of the spectrum.

	Point Score
1. *Do you have chronic back-ache?*	10
2. *Do you have generalized muscle pain, especially after exercise?*	10
3. *Do you suffer from muscle cramps, tremors or eyes flicking uncontrollably?*	10
4. *Do you have a tendency to pull muscles easily with exercise?*	10
5. *Do you have a tendency to nervousness/panic attacks?*	10
6. *Do you have cold, white fingers when it is cold (Raynaud's phenomenon)?*	10
7. *Do you have a history of kidney stones?*	10
8. *Are there problems with constipation?*	10
9. *Is there any history of irregular heartbeat?*	10
10. *Is there a history of high blood pressure?*	10
11. *Any problems with premenstrual symptoms?*	5
12. *Have you taken diuretic (water) tablets for any period of time?*	10
13. *Do you drink more than 3 units of alcohol daily?*	5

It is possible to score 120 points in this section (women) or 115 (men). Any score in excess of 40 points would indicate possible magnesium deficiency; in excess of 70 points would make this a virtual certainty. Any patient scoring high in this section should certainly have his or her magnesium levels estimated, either by red blood cell magnesium levels, sweat test and magnesium retention test, or a myothermogram (*see Chapter 9*).

The Management of the Individual Asthmatic

Thus, a comprehensive history, often facilitated by a questionnaire such as this, should direct a specialist in allergy, environmental and nutritional medicine into exploring the five main areas of causation related to asthma.

A heavy score in the food allergy/intolerance section, with very low scores in all the other sections, should lead to an elimination diet or intradermal skin testing and desensitization.

A high score in the biological inhalant section should lead to intradermal skin testing and probably desensitization. This desensitization can be augmented by strategies to reduce inhalants, such as house dust mite, with mattress enclosures, effective vacuum cleaning, liquid nitrogen, acarocide paints and so on. In the chemical sensitivity part of the questionnaire, high scoring should be followed by intradermal skin testing for suspected chemicals and avoidance, if possible, of the chemicals implicated. If this is not possible, neutralization treatment for the respective chemicals should be tried. Evaluation of nutrient levels prior to supplementation of nutrients to enhance the functioning of the various enzyme systems involved in detoxification should be considered.

If Candida hypersensitivity appears to be very important, an appropriate diet, as indicated in Chapter 8, plus anti-fungal medications should be considered. This treatment can take a month or two before a good result is obtained.

Magnesium deficiency, if confirmed with laboratory tests, should be corrected with magnesium supplements taken by mouth, although magnesium can be given by injection (intramuscularly or intravenously) if the condition is urgent enough.

Other nutritional strategies have been discussed in Chapter 9.

11

The Elimination Diet for Asthma

In Chapter 6 I discussed the theoretical side of the role of food allergy in asthma. In this chapter we get down to the practical side.

An elimination diet is an extremely educative experience for both doctor and patient, particularly the patient, who has first-hand experience during the course of this diet of how his or her body reacts to certain foods. At this point it should be emphasized that an elimination diet can lead to quite severe asthmatic reactions in patients who suffer from severe asthma, and such patients should only attempt an elimination diet under the guidance of a physician who is familiar with such diets and this type of patient. It should be emphasized, as has been discussed earlier, that food sensitivity plays a role for only some patients suffering from asthma, not all. I refer the reader at this point to Chapter 10, where it is pointed out that in some patients the problem is limited to inhaled allergens, such as dust, dust mites, moulds, chemicals and other airborne allergens, in some it is food sensitivity, and in others it is a bit of both. In those in whom it is a bit of both it is ideal to sort out the inhaled side of the problem by skin testing and neutralization prior to considering an elimination diet. If this is not done, food reactions can easily be confused with contacts with airborne allergens. Thus, if a patient has negative skin tests to aero-allergens and has been told that the asthma is intrinsic and relatively mild, then a 'do-it-yourself' elimination diet would be a very reasonable procedure.

As would be expected, some asthmatics find the diet very easy to follow, very acceptable and very easy to assess. Many patients find an improvement in excess of 90 per cent within seven days of starting the diet, with subsequent quite clear-cut reactions to a handful of foods. If these foods are then reasonably easy to avoid, the patient can do so and I have seen many asthmatics who have never needed to replace their existing supply of inhalers once this was done. Such patients are a delight to deal with and their whole attitude to their asthma changes completely. They know what is causing their problem, they no longer need medication, and this comes as a great relief to them (and to the public purse).

Other patients may find that their symptoms clear satisfactorily between six and eight days from starting the diet, but they then seem to react adversely to a huge range of foods, sometimes 15 to 20 separate items.

In the early days of conducting elimination diets, I found it difficult to accept that patients could react to so many different foods, but after many years and much re-testing of foods backed up by skin testing, I consider that most of these patients' observations have been quite genuine. People do not want to react adversely, particularly to their favourite foods, and there is probably more of a tendency to disregard minor reactions to favourite foods than to invent reactions that do not exist.

The most difficult cases are the small minority who have incredibly slow and insidious reactions to foods. Such people may take 12–24 hours to react to a food like milk, which most people will react to in less than 5 hours. If, in addition, they react to a large number of foods, then an elimination diet can be an extremely difficult, frustrating and highly unsatisfactory procedure. They may go for days or weeks trying to find a few foods that they appear to be all right with. Such people can, if they are not careful, run themselves into considerable nutritional difficulties, and when they relate their experience to a physician who is not familiar with the advantages and pitfalls of elimination diets, the physician may be somewhat dismayed at what they have done and adopt an extremely negative attitude to the whole concept.

Those whose symptoms clear nicely after the first few days of the Stage I diet, but who find themselves apparently reacting to a very large number of foods, should abandon the elimination diet and have their allergies sorted out by intradermal provocative skin testing. Certainly this would apply to someone reacting to four or five of the first six foods that are tried. My major reservations regarding the wisdom of detailing an elimination diet in this book concerns this very point. I know how determined some people become once they have seen their asthmatic symptoms improve without the benefit of drugs on the first stage of this diet.

It is important for a patient to select a good time to do an elimination diet, as it is a fairly anti-social procedure. Eating out, eating at other people's houses and so forth are virtually impossible in the first two or three weeks. There is, in fact, some difficulty but not impossibility in this respect for the whole eight weeks' duration (approximately) of the elimination diet. It is also a good idea to choose a time when maximum support can be obtained from people who are close to you and are concerned about the problem you are suffering.

Drugs

Many medications that are used in the control of asthma are taken in the form of tablets or capsules. Tablets, in particular, contain items such as corn starch and lactose (milk sugar), cane sugar and beet sugar. These foodstuffs are used as binding and filling agents and sugar-coatings. The standard way in which a pharmaceutical company will make up a tablet is to pour liquid corn starch or lactose into a mould and then add the active ingredients. All of these foods are common food allergens and this makes the use of these drugs hazardous in the first stage of the elimination diet. Normally, a little morsel of corn flour or lactose in tablets does not matter when the patient is eating those foods several times a day in other forms, but in the first stage of an elimination diet it does matter. Even a small amount of a food to which a patient is sensitive can have a profound effect, and the patient may not lose symptoms that would otherwise disappear.

The use of asthma inhalers, such as Ventolin, Atrovent, Duravent, Becotide, etc., causes no problem at all in this respect.

Steroids, such as Prednisolone and Betnosol, do contain corn starch in their standard form, but there is one formulation, Prednesol (Glaxo), which does not. Prednesol is designed to dissolve in water and contains no standard foodstuff. Five mg of Prednesol is exactly equivalent to 5 mg of Prednisolone.

Aside from drugs used to relieve or control asthma, some sufferers may be taking other drugs such as the contraceptive pill, sleeping tablets and blood pressure tablets. The contraceptive pill contains corn flour, etc., as do the other pills. Obviously the contraceptive pill must be continued until the end of a specific cycle; thereafter mechanical means of contraception should be used during the elimination procedure.

Sleeping tablets or capsules are a great problem for some. People often become very dependent on them and cannot sleep without them. If it is essential that you take them, one would hope that the small amount of corn starch involved would not affect the final result.

Blood pressure pills have to also be discontinued, at least temporarily, and your doctor told of this. I have never seen anyone's blood pressure rise on the first stage of this diet; very frequently it actually goes down, despite the withdrawal of these pills. The reason for this is that many blood pressure problems are connected with food sensitivity.

The Elimination Diet

We now come to the diet itself, and it starts with a few days on a very low-risk allergy diet, called by some an 'oligo antigenic' diet. Such a diet consists of a handful of foods which the patient rarely eats and which are known to pose a low risk of allergy. These foods are used simply to 'keep the wolf from the door' while the patient avoids all those foods which are likely to cause a problem. For asthma, the foods I would most frequently start with are as follows:

- lamb: Grilled lamb chops, roast lamb, cold lamb, lamb's liver, lamb's kidneys
- venison: Roast or grilled
- salmon, Cod, Trout, Mackerel: Grilled, fried or boiled; fresh or frozen (not tinned or smoked)
- pears
- avocados
- parsnips
- turnips
- swedes (rutabaga)
- celery
- chinese bean sprouts
- sweet potatoes (yams): These are very nice cut into penny slices and deep fried until brown, or microwaved into crisps.
- marrow
- courgette (zucchini)
- carrots.

For cooking, sunflower oil or safflower oil can be used.

If any of the above list is normally consumed more than two times a week, that food should be omitted from the diet.

Of course, vegetarians who wish to do this diet would have to omit the fish and the meat.

The only liquid which is allowed on the diet is one of the bottled spring waters, such as Malvern water, Evian, Perrier, Volvic, Highland Spring, etc. It does not appear to matter whether the water is still or sparkling, and this can be left to personal taste. Should the patient wish to liquidize the carrots or the pears with spring water and make a vegetable or fruit juice, this would be quite acceptable.

Pure sea salt can be used for flavouring the food.

It is to be emphasized that cigarette smoking should be totally discontinued on this diet. Anyone who smokes, as well as having asthma, is definitely asking for trouble. There is absolutely no doubt that cigarette smoking impairs lung function, partly by impairing the action of the small ciliary muscles in the bronchioles which cause the ciliary hairs to waft harmful substances out of the bronchiole tubes. Many asthmatics are also specifically sensitive to cigarette smoke, and what most do not appreciate is that cigarette tobacco is cured using sugar as part of what is known as the casing. Thus cigarette smoke can upset an elimination diet in several ways.

There remain three further pieces of advice which you should follow:

1. Sodium bicarbonate solution should be substituted for toothpaste, as various components of toothpaste can be absorbed under the tongue and cause problems.
2. Licking stamps and envelopes can cause problems, as the glue contains corn and several chemicals.
3. A large dose of Epsom salts should be taken on the first morning of the elimination diet to evacuate foods consumed on the days preceding the diet. Two teaspoons of Epsom salts are adequate for most adults, and one teaspoon for children over five years old. The Epsom salts should be dissolved in about ¼ pint of spring water.

It is to be emphasized that the above list of foods are the *only* foods that can be eaten on Stage I of this diet. There is, therefore, no tea, no coffee, no alcohol, no bread, no milk, no sugar, no eggs, etc. Many people find that breakfast is the most strange meal to have to cope with using these restrictions. For those who wish to have a snack, some pears, avocados, celery, carrots and sweet potatoes should suffice. There is, however, no reason why the patient should not have a cooked breakfast with one of the fish combined with one of the vegetables. The main meals of the day can be meat or fish, with plenty of root vegetables and marrow, finishing with some fruit.

Some people with very positive attitudes quite enjoy this diet and like the challenge it presents them with. If they also find their asthma rapidly disappearing, then the whole procedure is quite easy to endure.

Others can find the diet very trying. They feel upset that they cannot eat their bread, drink their tea, etc. They sometimes complain that they cannot face eating foods other than those which they are used to eating every day of their lives. They have what a close colleague of mine, Dr. Jonathan Maberly, has termed a 'grief reaction' for their 'lost foods'. Amazingly, such patients can arrive on the seventh day of the elimination diet showing enormous or total improvement in their asthma and still be quite unhappy because their diet is so restricted. They do not appear to appreciate the enormity of the fact that their symptoms have gone and that they are well on their way to discovering the cause of their problem.

What Happens on Stage I

At this point it is important to recall the whole concept of masking which was described in detail in Chapter 6. When patients go onto a diet such as has just been described, they should, if they have a masked food allergy, feel distinctly worse for the first three or four days of the diet. They are no longer obtaining the temporary lift that further doses of the allergenic food normally lead to. Thus, they are worse for the first few days of this diet for the same reason as the alcoholic is worse when he or she stops taking alcohol.

Classically, the afternoon/evening of the first day usually sees a distinct worsening of the asthma, and those who have discontinued their tablets or capsules which control their asthma may feel that this is quite normal and to be expected. However, it also occurs in those who normally control their asthma purely with inhalers, which of course they can still use. The afternoon/evening of the first day of the diet are frequently accompanied by a severe headache, if the patient is in any way prone to these. Should the patient normally suffer from migraine, that can virtually be guaranteed to occur on the first day, as migraine is almost always a food allergy problem.

The second day of the diet is usually a very bad day. The asthma is often quite bad and fatigue is frequently a marked feature. There may be some headache still remaining from the first day, and about 50 per cent of patients spend most of the second day in bed. At my clinic we often have a 'second day phone call' from concerned relatives who may not understand the logic of the withdrawal phenomenon.

The third day of the diet is sometimes as bad as the second day, and by now there may be depression coming into the clinical picture.

Some people may, however, notice some improvement in their asthma on this day.

However, the third day very frequently marks the onset of *withdrawal myalgia*, which is one of the classic features of the allergy withdrawal syndrome. Typically, muscle aches and pains occur in the lower back, buttocks and thighs. Sometimes these pains occur in other major muscle groups, such as the shoulders, arms, neck and lower legs. These pains are often quite severe on Days 3, 4 and 5, but usually ease on Days 6 and 7, although they occasionally go on to Days 8 or 9. These muscle pains are usually nothing to worry about, they are just a positive confirmation of the food allergy withdrawal syndrome.

The overriding concern in the latter part of the elimination diet is, however, to observe a large decrease in the tightness of the chest. If a patient's problems are food sensitivity, then the chest should be distinctly better after avoiding a food to which he or she is sensitive for at least six days.

The End of Stage I – Evaluation Day 7

This is the time to take stock of what has happened since the start of the diet. I always see patients under my care on this day. What I am predominantly concerned about on this day is how the patient feels in terms of his or her asthma. Those whose problems are exclusively food sensitivity usually rate themselves 80 – 90 per cent improved on this day.

If such an improvement has occurred, particularly with a characteristic story of withdrawal symptoms on the first few days of the diet, I am happy we are dealing with a food allergy problem. The contrast of the worst two or three days the patient has recently experienced followed two days later by the best two days is usually so marked that it is difficult to imagine it has occurred by chance.

Some people show virtually no withdrawal reaction at all. Their symptoms are the same as usual on Days 1–3, generally followed by a gradual improvement on Days 4, 5 and 6. I have no idea why this should occur, as they frequently turn out to have just the same sort of food allergies as those who suffer the classic withdrawal symptoms.

Another odd pattern I sometimes see is patients who follow the classic pattern until Day 6. Expecting to arise better than ever on Day 7, they awake to find their asthma has returned again in full force. Happily, these symptoms normally go away about 36 hours later. Sometimes this phenomenon, which I call an 'echo effect', occurs a bit later, on the evening of the seventh day after testing the first food on Stage II. The individuals will properly ascribe the recurrence of symptoms to that food, but on re-trial a week later, usually no reaction occurs. Why this echo effect occurs I have no idea, but similar things happen in classic immunology and there may one day be discovered a logical explanation for it.

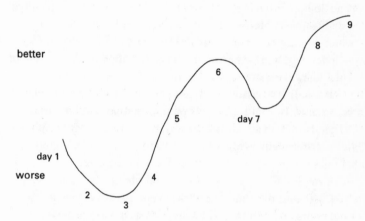

Figure 22 Withdrawal pattern followed by echo response

If, therefore, there is the satisfactory outcome of markedly improved lung function, the patient can now proceed to the second stage of the diet.

If There Is No Improvement

The most likely explanation is that food allergy is not an important part of that particular patient's asthma. It would suggest that airborne allergies, chemical sensitivity or the candida yeast problem is the real culprit. Thus, a flat response with no worsening in the first few days of the diet and no improvement would indicate that a change of direction is needed.

However, there is another pattern that has been observed in some patients. In these patients there is a classical withdrawal reaction in the first few days of the diet, followed by a return to the normal level of asthma and hence no improvement.

The fact that a withdrawal response has occurred would indicate that food sensitivity was important. The lack of improvement might indicate that the patient is, very unluckily, sensitive to a food on the low-risk diet. At my clinic, if we see this we skin test the patient to the Stage I foods to see if any of them are positive. However, if the patient is doing this diet unsupervised, it can be very difficult to know quite what is going wrong in these circumstances.

Stage II

The prime object of this stage is to expand the diet as quickly as possible. To that end we have selected, especially in the first three or four days, foods which are unlikely to give adverse reactions. There then follow foods which are generally desirable, but have only a moderate risk of allergy, plus a few that have fairly high risks. A suggested order of introduction follows. It is advisable to stick to this rigidly, as the safer foods are introduced earlier, and members of similar food families are separated by four days. This avoids the possibility of false negative responses through cross-reactivity within specific food families. Two foods are included for each day, starting with one food on the evening of Day 7, after the seventh-day evaluation. One food should be tested in the morning at breakfast time and one in the evening, thus allowing at least nine or ten hours between tests. This should be adequate time for reactions to these foods to develop. Lunchtime is limited to those foods that were on Stage I or which have already been passed as safe on Stage II. It does not matter on any particular day which of the two foods is tested in the morning and which in the evening.

Stage II Order of Food Reintroduction

Day 7 (evening)	broccoli
Day 8	green beans of any sort
	chicken
Day 9	spinach
	mushrooms
Day 10	brown rice
	bananas
Day 11	tap water
	black tea (whichever tea you normally consume)
Day 12	cow's milk (whole milk)
	grapes
Day 13	apples
	pork

Day 14	pure ground coffee
	leeks
Day 15	eggs
	melon
Day 16	beef
	yeast (brewer's yeast – 1 teaspoon) *possibly mixed with banana if banana test is satisfactory*
Day 17	butter
	cabbage

In the event of one of these foods being unavailable, fresh pineapple can be substituted on any day.

When testing food, the most important thing to watch for is, of course, the recurrence of asthma. However, if headache, fatigue or any other symptomatology that was part of the original problem recurs, it is sensible to regard this as a reaction, at least for the time being. Symptoms most commonly start within four to five hours, but nine to ten hours is left between tests to accommodate those who tend to react slowly.

Reactions to foods vary considerably in intensity, like everything in life. The big, bad reactions are exceedingly obvious to all patients. Before the reaction occurs the lungs are probably feeling very good, but within two or three hours of eating the allergic food, the patient can observe a marked recurrence of wheezing. The contrast of feeling so good followed within a few hours by feeling so bad is obvious. Other reactions are moderately obvious, but inevitably the situation sometimes arises when the patient is not sure.

This situation is particularly likely to occur when the patient is concurrently sensitive to airborne allergens, such as animal furs, dust, dust mite, etc. Despite neutralization, an unusually high exposure to such items may provoke some wheeze at the same time that the patient has introduced a new food. Is this a response to the food or the airborne allergen? There is only one way out of this dilemma, and that is to re-test the food. The ultimate saving grace of elimination diets is the ability to re-test.

On the day of the re-test the patient should make sure that there are no confusing variables such as mentioned above, which will confuse the issue again. However, the most important rule to obey is NEVER RE-TEST A FOOD WITHIN FIVE DAYS OF THE ORIGINAL TEST.

The only time that an immediate reaction to a food occurs is when it has been omitted from the diet for a minimum of five days. If it is omitted for a shorter period that this, a reaction will occur, but it will be delayed and possibly not associated with that food. Thus, the two major rules of food testing are:

1. If in doubt about a food reaction, leave the food out of the diet.
2. Never re-test a food in fewer than five days from the original test.

When a reaction to a food occurs, all the patient's asthmatic symptoms will flood back. The total duration of the reaction can be anything from 12 hours to four or five days, and during this time no food testing can be accomplished. The patient should therefore restrict him- or herself to those foods already found to be safe, until the symptoms pass. This, of course, slows ups the testing programme, and all the timing of reintroducing foods on certain days changes. To speed up the clearing of a reaction, the following mixture is strongly recommended:

2 teaspoons sodium bicarbonate
1 teaspoon potassium bicarbonate

These two bicarbonates are placed in ¼ pint (140 ml) of hot water and stirred until dissolved. The sodium bicarbonate is ordinary bicarbonate of soda, which is obtainable at any pharmacy or supermarket. The potassium bicarbonate can be quite difficult to obtain. However, pharmacists should be able to obtain it from a wholesaler.

The mixture is pretty revolting to take, and most people prefer to swallow it in one gulp. It usually does two things:

1. It should lead to a bowel movement, and the allergic food tends to be eliminated from the intestines. Clearly, the faster this occurs, the better.
2. Food reactions are accompanied by a reactionary acidosis: all body fluids become slightly more acid, and this indirectly causes many of the symptoms. A large dose of alkali (the two bicarbonates) corrects this situation to some extent.

Lately, at my clinic we have been using an improved version of this combination which is called 'Turn-Off' Food Allergy Treatment. In the UK it is produced by a firm called Allergy Care (Pollards Yard, Wood Street, Taunton, Somerset, TA1 1UT). The formulation is similar to that described above, but it has malik acid added and is considerably more palatable. The makers suggest a dosage of one level teaspoon, but we find most people require nearer two level teaspoons if they are adults. The medication is inexpensive.

These sodium/potassium bicarb mixtures, therefore, act in two separate and complementary ways. A single dose of this mixture will normally halve the reaction time. A further dose can be taken up to about six hours later, if necessary. When the symptoms have subsided for a couple of hours, further testing can commence.

At the end of Stage II there should be a general review of what has occurred. It is hoped that there will have been a substantial improvement in the symptoms by the end of Stage I, followed by a maintenance of that improvement for most of Stage II. Individuals who have only two or three food sensitivities may negotiate the whole of Stage II without reaction.

The main question to ask at this point concerns how much improvement has been obtained between any reactions to foods. If there is 90 – 100 per cent improvement between reactions on Stage II, then the problems are almost certainly exclusively food sensitivity. If there is only, for example, a 30 – 70 per cent improvement, there is probably an inhaled component to the problems. This may be either a chemical problem such as a gas, or one of the common inhaled allergens such as dust, dust mite, mould or animal dander. To sort these out a competent allergist, familiar with this approach, is usually needed.

There are 21 foods in Stage II. Quite a lot of people will react to five or six of these foods, and such individuals will normally end up with about 12–16 food sensitivities by the end of Stage IV. These people will eventually, almost certainly, need neutralization therapy to enable them to eat relatively normally in the long run. Any person reacting to something like 15 or more of the 21 foods should immediately resort to the intradermal skin testing and neutralization approach. Should there be a delay before this type of help can be obtained, it is probably best to resume a normal diet, plus your original drugs, in the intervening time.

Stage III

This stage contains many common food allergens, including the cereals, which need special consideration in their testing. Cereals, especially wheat, are very slowly absorbed and most frequently take 36 hours to produce a reaction. I have seen some patients even take over two days to react to wheat, and this, therefore, must be taken into account.

I have delayed testing potatoes and tomatoes until Stage III, as it appears that in some patients it can take over two weeks to get rid of the reactions to these foods from the solenacia family (which also includes deadly nightshade).

Day 18	potatoes
	oranges
Day 19, 20 & 21	Wheat

Test pure shredded wheat. The pure wheat should be eaten at all meals on these three days (plus all safe foods). The reaction to this foodstuff is not only slow to materialize, but if it occurs it is very slow to eradicate. I have seen some patients take four to five days before they feel well again.

Day 22	wholemeal bread

This should only be tested if both the wheat test and the yeast test are satisfactory. Try wholemeal bread at each meal for this day.

Day 23	onion
	tomatoes
Day 24	cane sugar

This is Jamaican, Trinidad or other West Indian demerara sugar. Muscovada is also satisfactory. Two teaspoons of cane sugar should be taken three times a day for one full day.

Day 25	prawns or shrimps
	peanuts

The peanuts should be obtained loose from a health food shop. Do not use the packaged variety, which have additives.

Day 26	beet sugar

This is retailed under the name of Silver Spoon in the UK. Usually it is pure beet sugar, but sometimes, if the beet sugar crop is inadequate in quantity, there can be a little cane sugar added. Allergies to cane sugar and beet sugar are quite separate, as they come from totally different plants. Please note: Tate & Lyle sugar has both cane and beet sugar in most samples. Spend one day on testing beet sugar, taking two teaspoons at each meal.

Day 27 & 28	corn

This very commonly consumed food should be tested in two forms: (1) corn on the cob, and (2) pure glucose powder. Glucose retailed in Britain is nearly always made from corn, although most retail chemists are unaware of this. Start each meal with corn on the cob (or loose) and finish the meal with two teaspoons of glucose. Take both forms of corn at each meal for two full days. Some people appear to react more obviously to one form of corn, and some to the other. Either way the reaction is to corn. Reactions to corn are slow but usually not quite as slow as to wheat; I have not seen them starting longer than 48 hours after commencing this test.

Day 29	lettuce
	soya beans (can be tested as pure soya milk)

Soy is very important. It is present in soya-bean oil (vegetable oils), soya-bean flour, etc. One way or another it is present in a huge range of manufactured foods.

Day 30	Cheddar cheese
	bacon (if pork is satisfactory)

When testing for bacon one is, in fact, testing for the nitrites and nitrate chemicals that are present in bacon. Check that there is no sugar mentioned on the labelling.

End of Stage III Assessment

Most patients will have reacted to at least one food by now. The Western diet is predominantly based on wheat, corn, cane sugar, beet sugar, yeast, milk, eggs, soy and potatoes. These main foods have now all been tested, and usually at this point the patient will have a shrewd idea of his or her problems. Otherwise, the comments I made on the Stage II assessment apply equally at this stage.

Stage IV

The object of Stage IV is to tidy up all the loose ends. If reactions to Stage II foods started within five hours, then three foods a day can now be tested (except for the remaining cereals). If not, continue to test two foods a day.

Day 31	white bread – (do not test if you are allergic to wheat, yeast, or corn)
	This is a test for chemicals, especially anti-staling agents which are present in white bread retailed in the UK.
Day 32	peas (if frozen, check no mint or sugar is added)
	grapefruit
	pure honey
Day 33	cucumber
	plaice
	black pepper (condiment pepper)
Day 34 & 35	rye

Use Ryvita (the original rye crispbread). Take rye at every meal for two full days unless a reaction occurs earlier. Test the pale variety of crispbread and not the dark variety, which also contains malt. If there is a reaction to rye and also to wheat, I do not think it is worthwhile testing oats or malt later, as reactions to these will by now be a foregone conclusion. If the wheat test is positive, but rye is negative, it is still wise to eat rye rather cautiously. Rye and wheat are very closely related in the botanical tables, and many people who are allergic to wheat will soon sensitize themselves to rye if they eat a lot of it. This is the most common cause of confusion and dismay on the last part of the elimination diet.

Day 36	instant coffee

Test Nescafé Gold Blend. This is another chemical test, testing for the preserving chemicals. Only test instant coffee if no reaction to ground coffee. Caution – many cheap instant coffees contain corn.

	asparagus
	lemon
Day 37	dry white wine

Test if no reaction to grapes or yeast. If there is a reaction to dry white wine then the reaction will be to sulphites. Sulphites are present in all wines, but most French and Australian wines contain quite a lot of sulphite. Therefore, ideally test wines from these countries.

	lentils
	canned carrots

*Do not test canned carrots if you are sensitive to carrots! The
object of this test is to test the phenolic resin lining of cans.
These linings are present in many tins, and canned carrots are
selected as a convenient sample. You should check that the can
contains no sugar if allergic to cane sugar, beet sugar or
glucose.*

Day 38   monosodium glutamate
*This is a flavour-enhancer used in many canned foods, sauces,
gravies, etc. It can be obtained in pure white crystalline form
in many supermarkets (especially Chinese and delicatessens).
A little of the powder should be sprinkled like salt over some
meat or almost any other foodstuff you prefer.*
turkey
brussels sprouts

Day 39 & 40   oats
*Ideally take porridge oats at every meal for two days or until a
reaction occurs.*

Day 41   saccharin (Sweetex drops)
red/green peppers
mixed herbs

Day 42   raisins (do not test if sensitive to grapes. This is a test for
Sulphur Dioxide which is blown over grapes during the
production of raisins.)
tartrazine yellow
*This is the yellow dye obtainable at most delicatessens. The
most commonly obtainable one is the yellow dye used for
making food mixtures like cakes, etc. Put two drops in about
10 drops of water and swill around the mouth.*

Day 43   cauliflower
chocolate
*Chocolate contains wheat, corn, and sugar – do not test if you
are allergic to any of these. Bitter chocolate is the same but
does not contain wheat.*

Day 44   olive oil
sodium benzoate

Day 45   malt
*Test for one full day – take two teaspoons of malt extract at
every meal (caution – some malt extracts contain wheat).*

End of Stage IV Assessment

By the end of this stage the average person will have assessed over 80 foods, which accounts for over 97 per cent of what most people eat. Fruits, such as cherries, plums, peaches, raspberries, gooseberries and blackcurrants are, of course, seasonal in their fresh form and have not been included in this elimination procedure, which has been devised to be used at any time of the year. These fruits should be tested when they become available in their normal season. None of them is a common food allergen.

Complicated manufactured foods, such as jams, confectionery, sauces, cakes, biscuits, gravies, pizzas and alcoholic beverages are mostly mixtures of items already tested, such as sugar, wheat, corn, yeast, soy and egg. If the patient suffers with this type of sensitivity, there will be problems with many manufactured foods, unless he or she has densensitization treatment. These foods may also contain many of the chemicals which have been tested, such as anti-staling agents, monosodium glutamate, saccharin, sulphites, sulphur dioxide, tartrazine yellow and sodium benzoate.

Lists of 'multiple foods' containing corn, wheat, yeast, milk, eggs and soy can be found at the end of this chapter. There is also an illustration (Figure 23) showing the common constituents of various alcoholic beverages and a dissertation on the role of alcohol (*see below*).

At the end of Stage IV the patient should, therefore, have what is perhaps best termed a 'compatible diet'. Most people will have found that, of the 80 items tested, 70 or more are satisfactory. On the face of it this sounds quite nice, but very frequently the 10 foods that are implicated are among the most difficult ones to avoid. For people who have to eat out a lot in the course of their occupation, neutralization is virtually essential. For those who eat mostly at home, avoidance may be a practical consideration, particularly if they can find less commonly eaten foods to substitute for foods such as wheat. Items such as buckwheat, buckwheat flour, sago, tapioca and chick-pea flour can be useful in this context. There are, of course, many excellent foods not tested on the above 80-food test regime, but anyone who has been through this regime will now know how to go about food testing, and any of these foods can now be tested and added to the repertoire.

Alcohol

A lot of asthma sufferers notice that the consumption of certain alcoholic beverages will almost certainly lead to a major flare-up of their asthma. This is, incidentally, a very positive indicator that food sensitivity is an important factor in the causation of these individuals' asthmatic reaction.

In the late 1940s Dr. Theron Randolph made a considerable intuitive leap in realizing that these reactions to alcoholic beverages resulted from the constituents of the drink and not the alcohol itself. What makes the reaction so obvious to many people is the rapid absorption. Everyone is familiar with the promptly observable effect of, for example, four double scotches consumed in quick succession. The main constituent of scotch whisky is grain, which when consumed normally, for example in the form of bread, takes many hours to be absorbed in any quantity. In the form of scotch whisky it is absorbed in a few minutes. Part of the reason for this rapid absorption is that, whereas food is normally absorbed only in the intestines, alcohol is absorbed throughout the whole intestinal tract, starting from the mouth, going through the stomach and duodenum and into the intestines. Dr. Randolph coined the phrase that reactions to alcoholic beverages represent 'food allergy in a jet-propelled vehicle'.

Most of the alcoholic drinks are derived from foods such as wheat, corn, cane sugar, grapes and potatoes. These items represent the more common food allergens. Remembering the concept of masking, it is obvious that to a wheat-allergic patient, an alcoholic drink containing wheat will have a quicker masking effect than were the wheat to be eaten conventionally, because of the rapid absorption. Hence, if allergy to wheat can lead to addiction to wheat, addiction to whisky will follow if the drinker is not careful. Alcoholism has been termed 'the acme of food allergy', and there is no doubt in my mind, having dealt with a number of alcoholics, that this is true. Sometimes, however, the rapidity of the absorption of the alcohol drink is such that it 'breaks through the masking process' and can give the patient a direct reaction to the food rather than produce a masking effect.

Conversely, if the alcoholic beverage contains a substance – for example grapes or a resin or a preserving chemical – which is not regularly present in the drinker's diet, then there may well be an unmasked hyper-acute reaction, made even more acute by the rapidity of absorption.

Always present = ˋ Sometimes present = O	Corn	Wheat, Barley, Rye*	Oats	Rice	Potatoes	Grapes	Plum	Citrus	Cherry	Apples	Hops	Juniper	Cinnamon	Mint	Miscellaneous Herbs	Cactus	Beet sugar	Cane sugar
Blended Scotch whisky	ˋ	ˋ															O	O
Malt Scotch whisky	O	ˋ															O	O
Canadian Blended whiskey	ˋ	ˋ				ˋ	ˋ	O									O	ˋ
Irish whiskey		ˋ	ˋ															O
Blended Irish whiskey	ˋ	ˋ	ˋ		ˋ	ˋ	O									O	O	
Gin (grain)	ˋ	ˋ	O	O				ˋ				ˋ	O	O	ˋ		O	O
Gin (cane) High & Dry												ˋ	ˋ	ˋ	ˋ			ˋ
Vodka	O	O			O												ˋ	ˋ
Jamaican rum																		ˋ
Tequila																ˋ		ˋ
Beer	O	ˋ	O	ˋ							ˋ							
Grape brandy	O					ˋ											O	O
Cordials & Liqueurs	ˋ	ˋ	O	O	O	ˋ	ˋ	ˋ	ˋ	ˋ			ˋ	ˋ	ˋ		ˋ	ˋ
Grape wine	O					ˋ											ˋ	ˋ
Sherry	ˋ					ˋ											ˋ	ˋ
Champagne						ˋ											O	O
Cider	ˋ									ˋ							ˋ	ˋ
Vermouth	O	O	O			ˋ											ˋ	ˋ
Cognac						ˋ											O	O
Cherry brandy	O								ˋ								O	O

*Please note that yeast occurs in all alcoholic beverages.

Figure 23

The law does not require that the contents of alcoholic drinks be stated on the bottle, and in general they are allowed to remain a trade secret. However, as a result of discussions with representatives of some major alcoholic manufacturers, it is possible to put together a rough guide to the content of the major alcoholic drinks obtainable in the UK. Most of the information presented in Figure 23 relates predominantly to products from the Distillers Corporation, the major supplier of alcoholic drinks in Britain. Vodkas, for example, can be made from a very wide range of foods, and some vodkas are made from potatoes, but a high proportion are now made from grains, especially wheat. Much of the information presented here was subsequently verified by patients with known food sensitivities who have managed to observe which alcoholic drinks they can tolerate and which they cannot.

It must be added that wines may contain a number of chemicals which are not mentioned in this list. The cheaper wines, particularly those imported in bulk, will normally have chemicals added to them to stop them deteriorating while travelling. As most travellers know, cheap wines do not travel well in the normal course of events, and so preserving chemicals have to be added to maintain them in good condition. Reaction to these chemicals is extremely prevalent and accounts, I think, for the common observation that cheap wine can cause a nasty hangover, whereas more expensive wine may well not. The severe hangover which some people may experience with certain alcoholic drinks is, in my opinion, usually because of specific food sensitivities occurring in those particular drinks. A more comprehensive review of this subject is given by Dr. Theron G. Randolph in the book entitled *Clinical Ecology* (Charles C. Thomas, 1976).

Foods Not Included in the Elimination Diet

There is a huge range of foods which it would be absurd to include in a standard elimination diet because many patients have never eaten them or eat them so rarely that they can't really be a problem. However, there is a wide variety of foods which people do eat – I have, for example, one patient who used to eat Macadamia nuts every day of his life and in his case it would clearly be important to test that food. I include, therefore the following list of 114 foods which, while not included in the elimination diet outlined above, may need to be tested by those patients who normally eat them regularly.

Vegetables (27)
alfalfa
artichokes
aubergines
bamboo shoots
beans, various:
    including aduki,
    broad (fava),
kidney, better (lima)
garden cress
gherkins
peas (various)
inc: black-eyed
    chick-peas
    (garbanzo)
    split
    cream
pumpkin
radishes
sago palm
salsify
squashes (various)
tapioca
watercress
yams
beansprouts
celeriac
chicory
kelp
okra

Fowl (7)
duck
goose
grouse
guinea fowl
pheasant
pigeon
quail

Meats (3)
rabbit
hare
venison

Nuts (10)
almonds
Brazil nuts
cashew nuts
chestnuts
filberts
hazelnuts
macadamia nuts
pecans
pistachios
walnuts

Grains (4)
barley
buckwheat
millet
wild rice

Fruits (24)
apricots
blackberries
blueberries
cantaloupe
cherries
clementines
crab apples
cranberries
elderberries
gooseberries
kiwi fruit
limes
loganberries
mandarins
mangoes
nectarines

pomegranates
plums
prunes
raspberries
satsumas
strawberries
tangerines
ugli fruit

Shellfish (8)
cockles
crab
lobster
mussels
oysters
scallops
whelks
winkles

Salt & Freshwater Fish (24)
anchovies
brill
bream
carp
caviar
eel
haddock
hake
halibut
huss
monkfish
mullet
perch
salmon
sardines
sea bass
sea herring
sole
squid/octopus

swordfish	*Miscellaneous (7)*	rhubarb
tunafish	herbal tea	arrowroot
turbot	green tea	China tea
whitebait	goat's milk	
whiting	sheep's milk	

This list of 114 foods does not contain the enormous range of individual herbs and spices which is available. Nor does it include many occasionally available foods. Various exotic fish and tropical fruits, for example, are now available in markets and restaurants.

All these foods are individual biological entities. As such they may not be tolerated by sufferers with complex food allergy problems. In people who have a simple food allergy problem of three or four commonly-eaten foods, they are all likely to be tolerated well.

These foods can gradually be reintroduced into the diet at the patient's leisure. Many people, especially those with very conservative eating habits, will probably eat hardly any of these items prior to a food allergy investigation. The general attitude of doctors in this field is to encourage their patients to eat as wide a range of foods as possible. As allergy seems frequently to relate to the frequency of ingestion of specific foods, the less frequently any individual food is consumed, the more likely the patient is to remain tolerant to it. To prevent the development of further food sensitivities, therefore, it is advisable to eat as wide a range of foods as possible. Many patients, when they first attend my clinic, tell me proudly that they eat very simply and never vary their diet. They consider this to be a virtue, but they are in fact wrong and it is probably one of the reasons why they need to attend my clinic in the first place.

Cheeses

Cheeses present a distinct problem on elimination diets. Obviously, if the cheese is manufactured partly from cow's milk and you are allergic to this, it is likely (but not certain) that you will react to the cheese. Cheeses are complex mixtures of foods and, as their constituents are trade secrets, it is very difficult to obtain a list like the one for alcohol (Figure 23). The 'Cheese Regulations' available from the UK Ministry of Agriculture, Fisheries and Food is not a lot of help in this respect, in that it just lists items that are permitted in certain cheeses. The best solution really is to try out the cheeses individually after the main exclusion diet has been completed. Cheeses commonly tried include Bel Paese, Brie, Camembert, Cheshire, cottage Cheese, Edam, Emmenthal, Gorgonzola, Gouda, Gruyère, Parmesan, Roquefort, Stilton and Swiss. Cheddar cheese has been evaluated on the original diet.

Foods Containing Wheat

Bread
Biscuits
Canned and frozen foods (some)
Cereal-derived sauces
Cheese spreads containing cereal products as fillers
Chocolate (all except bitter chocolate)
Coffee substitutes
Commercial cakes
Commercial salad dressings made with wheat flour
Crackers made from wheat
Flour
Gravies
Ice cream
Ice cream cones
Luncheon meats
Macaroni
Malt
Meat loaf
Meat or fish rissoles
Noodles
Pastas
Oatmeal (some)
Ovaltine
Pancakes
Pastries and pies
Puddings
Sausages
Any sauce or gravy thickened with wheat flour
Soups thickened with wheat flour
Spaghetti
Tortillas
Vermicelli
Waffles
Various alcoholic drinks
Most beers, whiskies and gins

Foods Containing Corn

Adhesives (envelopes, stamps, stickers)
Bacon (some)
Baking mixtures
Baking powders
Batters
Biscuits
Bleached wheat flour
Breads and pastries (some)
Cakes
Canned fruits (some)
Canned peas
Carbonated beverages (most)
Cheeses (some)
Chilli
Chocolate
Coated rice
Cornflakes
Cough syrups
Cream pies
Custards
Dates (sweetened)
Deep fat frying mixtures

Frozen fruits (some)
Fruit juices (some)
Gelatin desserts
Glucose products
Grape juice (some)
Gravies
Gum
Hams (some)
Ice cream
Icing sugar
Inhalants (bath and body powders)
Instant coffee (some)
Instant teas (some)
Jams
Jellies
Milk in paper cartons
Margarine
Peanut butter
Popcorn
Preserves
Puddings
Salad dressings

Sandwich spreads
Sauces
Sherbets
Soups
Soya milks (some)
Starch (cornflour)
String beans – canned and frozen (some)
Sweeteners
Sweets
Syrups
Tortillas
Vanilla
Vegetables – canned and frozen (some)
Vinegar (some)
Most tablets, capsules, lozenges, suppositories

Alcohol: most beers, whiskies, gins, sherries, cheap wines (*see Figure 23*)

Foods Containing Milk or Milk Products
Au gratin foods (potatoes, beans)
Baker's bread
Baking powder biscuits
Boiled salad dressings
Bologna
Butter
Buttermilk
Butter sauces
Cakes
Candies
Cheese
Chocolate or cocoa drinks
Chowders

Cream
Creamed foods
Cream sauces
Curd
Custards
Doughnuts
Eggs, scrambled
Gravy
Hamburger buns
Junket
Ice cream
Malted milk
Margarine
Mashed potatoes
Meat loaf

Milk, condensed, dried,	Omelettes
evaporated, powdered)	Quiche
Mixes for:	Rarebits
biscuits	Salad dressings
cakes	Sherbets
doughnuts	Soda Crackers
muffins	Soufflés
pancakes	Soups
pie crust	Waffles
puddings	Whey
waffles	Yogurt

Foods Containing Yeast

1. Foods that contain yeast as an additive:
   Biscuits
   Breads
   Cakes and cake mix
   Flour enriched with yeast vitamins
   Foods dried in breadcrumbs
   Hamburgers
   Hot dog rolls
   Milk fortified with vitamins from yeast
   Pastries
   Pretzels
2. The following substances contain yeast or yeast-like substances because of their nature or the nature of their manufacture or preparation:
   Mushrooms, truffles, cheeses of all kinds, buttermilk, and cottage cheese.
   Various vinegars, such as apple, pear, grape, and distilled vinegar. These vinegars can also occur in mayonnaise, olives, pickles, sauerkraut, condiments, horseradish, French dressings, salad dressings, barbecue sauce, tomato sauce, chilli peppers, and mince pies.
   All alcoholic drinks – whiskies, gins, wines, brandy, rum, vodka, beer, etc.
   Malted products: cereals, sweets, chocolates, and milk drinks which have been malted.
   Citrus fruit juices, either frozen or canned. Almost all commercial citrus fruit juices contain yeast.

3. Many vitamin products are derived from yeast or have their sources in yeast.

Foods Containing Soya Beans
1. Bakery goods
   Soya bean flour containing only 1 per cent of oil is now used by some bakeries in their dough mixtures for breads, rolls, cakes and pastries. This keeps them moist and saleable several days longer. The roasted nuts are used in place of peanuts.
2. Sauces
   Oriental soya sauce
   Lea & Perrins Sauce
   La Choy Sauce
   Heinz Worcestershire Sauce
3. Salad dressing
   Many salad dressings and mayonnaises contain soya oil, but only state on the label that they contain vegetable oil.
4. Meats
   Pork sausage and luncheon meats may contain soya beans.
5. Sweets
   Soya flour is used in hard sweets. Lecithin is invariably derived from soya beans and is used in sweets to prevent drying out, and to emulsify the fats.
6. Milk substitutes
   Some bakers use soya milk instead of cow's milk.
7. Ice cream
8. Soups
9. Vegetables
   Fresh soya sprouts are served as a vegetable, especially in Chinese dishes.
10. Soya nuts are roasted, salted, and used instead of peanuts.
11. Soya bean noodles, macaroni, and spaghetti.
12. Margarine and butter substitutes.

How to Desensitize to Inhaled Allergens

Desensitization by the neutralization technique is the key to much of the successful management of asthma, as the reader may have noted from the case histories described in Chapter 4.

Although major improvements can be achieved, for example by modification of the indoor air environment such as described in Chapter 5, these modifications will only improve things while the patient is within his or her own home environment.

But housedust, dust mites, moulds, animal danders and so forth will also exist in schools, other people's houses and in the workplace. Atmospheric moulds and pollens are impossible to avoid, usually short of emigration to a very hot, dry climate, preferably a desert clime with virtually no vegetation. Some mild asthmatics may find modifications to their home will so reduce their 'total load' that they can cope with other exposures without major problems. However, this is not good enough for the moderately severe or very severe asthmatics, in whose case neutralization is really the solution.

After neutralization treatment commences, most patients notice a marked improvement within a few days. Maximum improvement is attained, usually, within two to three weeks. With inhaled allergies, neutralizing injections or neutralizing sublingual drops are needed for about 15 months before complete desensitization is achieved. In the case of injections they need to be self-administered on alternate days, and in the case of the sublingual (under the tongue) drops, administration is needed three times a day. Most people are a little bit worried about the prospect of giving themselves an injection, but the needles are microfine and almost impossible to feel. We have found self-injection to be an entirely acceptable solution for at least 95 per cent of patients, and this is the experience of several thousand other physicians scattered around the world.

Now, the word 'cure' is a pretty emotive one and most doctors are rather shy of using it. However, if after 15 months of neutralizing injections or sublingual drops, a patient has no sign of asthma and is taking no medication at all, I think the word can be fairly applied. Physicians working in this field have seen countless patients where this scenario has occurred.

The Discovery of the Phenomenon of Neutralization

Allergists who have worked for years giving patients arbitrary and increasing doses of injected allergens for inhaled allergy problems (the old-fashioned incremental desensitization) have known that an occasional patient here and there would report a startling improvement in his or her condition within an hour or so of receiving an allergy injection. This improvement would often last for a few days. Such patients would often return and ask for a further injection 'exactly the same as the last one'. This rapid relief phenomenon, which flew totally in the face of conventional theory, puzzled most allergists. It was considered by most to be a psychological quirk. However, in 1957 Dr. Carleton H. Lee of Missouri made the discovery which on the one hand explained this curious phenomenon, but on the other opened up the most amazing vistas for the control of allergic responses to inhaled allergens as well as to foods, chemicals and even hormones and viruses.

Dr. Lee's wife had severe asthma which he had discovered was related to the consumption of certain common foods. Unfortunately she reacted to a huge range of foods and could remain well on only two or three specific foods. Other foods would quickly bring on moderate or severe asthmatic attacks within a few hours.

Although food extract injection therapy had never before been found to have had any use, Dr. Lee persisted in experimenting with injecting food extracts in the hopes of helping his wife's problem. He eventually discovered to his delight that he could produce asthmatic symptoms with one carefully measured dose of food extract injected intradermally (between the layers of the skin). More importantly, he found that another specific concentration would relieve this asthma within 10 minutes. This specific dose became known as 'the neutralizing dose'. He then went on to observe that this specific dose, when given by a small subcutaneous injection (just under the skin), would protect his wife for the next two or three days should she eat that particular food. A cocktail of all the neutralizing doses of the foods to which she was sensitive, administered in a single injection about three times a week, would enable her to eat normally without any asthma.

Thus was born provocation neutralization testing and treatment. The word provocation refers to the production of symptoms with one dose of the injected allergen. The term neutralization relates to the relief of symptoms with another dose. Neutralization therapy is the treatment of the problem with low, tailor-made doses of the allergen, usually and most effectively administered by subcutaneous injection. Administration can also be effected with sublingual (under the tongue) drops, which we will discuss later.

Soon Dr. Lee discovered that he could utilize the same principles to 'neutralize' reactions to inhaled allergens such as housedust, dust mites, moulds, animal furs and summer pollens. It had been possible to treat such problems before with conventional incremental desensitization, but the success rate was low (often below 20 per cent) and the treatment took months or years to work. The relief with inhaled allergen neutralizing injections often starts within half an hour of the first neutralizing injection being administered, and lasts for several days.

Safety

In 1986 in Great Britain, desensitization treatment suddenly made the headlines in the national press. The Committee on Safety in Medicine, a Government-appointed watchdog on the pharmaceutical industry, suddenly ruled that conventional incremental desensitization should only be administered by doctors working in units where there was adequate resuscitative equipment and the knowledge to use it. Furthermore, they ruled that patients were to remain in the units for an hour or so until it was quite certain that no very adverse response to the injection had occurred.

Up to the time of this ruling most of the incremental desensitizing injections had been given rather casually at the doctor's, and often the patient had been allowed to go home immediately. Many doctors had not been well trained in how to deal with the adverse allergic reactions that these injections often initiated. As a result of this there had been over the previous few years a handful of patients who had died as a direct result of this type of treatment. Most of these patients were severe asthmatics, who are, in any case, amongst the most difficult patients to handle in the whole field of allergic practice.

As a result of this ruling incremental desensitization virtually stopped in the UK, except in a few allergy units in National Health Service hospitals. Although the safety of incremental desensitization was probably much higher than that of many drugs still used, such as the anti-inflammatory drugs used by the million for treating arthritis, the benefit/risk ratio was low. Risks with a specific treatment are often tolerated if the potential benefits of that treatment are high. The potential benefits, however, of incremental desensitization are very low. Only about 15 per cent of patients benefit from desensitization to allergens such as housedust, dust mite and moulds. The success rate with desensitization to summer pollens is greater, but because the season is limited, summer problems are usually less of a strain on patients than allergens which affect them all year round, such as housedust.

In total contrast, with provocative neutralization therapy we observe almost total safety. There has not to my knowledge been a single fatality recorded anywhere in the world as a result of provocative neutralization therapy or testing. Currently there are only about 15 clinics using this method in the UK. There are, however, over 4,000 clinics in the US using this technique. Provocative neutralization is used as the method of choice by members of the American Academy of Environmental Medicine, the American Academy of Otolaryngolic Allergy and the Pan American Allergy Society. The combined membership of these large societies exceeds over 3,000 physicians, and all these societies run annual instructional courses for physicians interested in the technique.

In the UK my clinic pioneered provocative neutralization testing starting in 1977, but many American clinics had been using it for years prior to this. Dr. Lee made his initial observations in 1957 and treated many patients in the years after this. Dr. Joseph Miller became interested in 1965 and had gained so much experience in it over the next few years that in 1972 he published his book, *Food Allergy: Provocative Testing and Injection Therapy*. This became the 'bible' for many other American allergists, who started treating patients in this manner soon after. In 1987, Dr. Miller published a major tome on the subject entitled, *Relief at Last: Neutralization for Food Allergy and Other Illnesses*. Also in 1987, Dr. Carleton H. Lee published a definitive book about his technique entitled *Allergy Neutralization: The Lee Method*. This book further extended our knowledge of Dr. Lee's enormous ingenuity.

At least 20 million patients, at a conservative estimate, have therefore received this form of treatment over a period of many years without any fatalities. Most of these patients were in the US or Canada, but many thousands have also been treated in the UK and Australia.

This safety factor is not surprising when one considers that the provocation neutralization method uses doses that are frequently several thousand times weaker than those used in incremental desensitization. Furthermore, the tailor-made doses employed for neutralization are ones which:

a) have a completely negative skin reaction
b) have an immediate positive health benefit.

In 1987 the UK Committee on Safety in Medicine, in a letter to Dr. Jean Monro, acknowledged that their strictures concerning incremental desensitization did not apply to low-dose neutralization therapy, which they had not considered in their deliberations.

The Technique

Inhaled allergen extracts of housedust, dust mite, various moulds, various animal danders, feathers, wool, various summer pollens and so on are obtained in standard 1-in-10 or 1-in-20 prick test solutions. These concentrates need to be diluted to various strengths, and the dilutant that most clinics use nowadays is triple-distilled normal saline, containing a small amount of benzyl alcohol to ensure sterility. Many years ago we used to use phenol for this purpose, but some patients were sensitive to the phenol itself, so we switched to benzyl alcohol which has a very low incidence of allergy or potential for sensitization. Using this dilutant of saline/benzyl alcohol, we prepare nine separate solutions of, for example, dust mite. The strongest dilution is a 1-in-5 solution and is called the number 1.

Number 1 dilution	=	1/5 solution
Number 2 dilution	=	1/25 solution
Number 3 dilution	=	1/125 solution
Number 4 dilution	=	1/625 solution
Number 5 dilution	=	1/3125 solution
and so on.		

The testing procedure involves giving intradermal (between the layers of the skin) injections of these various concentrations of any allergens which are suspected in each individual case.

The logistics of sorting out inhaled allergy, therefore, fall into two categories:

1. sorting out which airborne allergens are likely to be affecting the patient
2. obtaining the right neutralizing levels to each of these allergens.

The response to an intradermal injection of inhaled allergen is determined 10 minutes after it is originally given. Assessing whether this wheal is positive or negative is the whole crux of a successful or unsuccessful outcome to this procedure, and allergy medicine professionals go through extensive training to ensure that they are able to distinguish between positive and negative wheals.

When 1/20th of a cc of an inhalant extract is injected intradermally it will, at the time of injection, produce a wheal which is hard, raised, blanched and has well-demarcated edges. The wheal will normally measure about 6mm × 6mm or 7mm × 7mm. After 10 minutes a positive wheal will usually have retained most of these features and will have grown by at least 2mm in diameter. Negative wheals lose these characteristics and grow by less than 2mm. If the initial injection results in a positive wheal, with or without symptoms, the practitioner moves to consecutively weaker strengths until the first negative wheal is discovered. This is the neutralizing dose and also the treatment concentration, unless symptoms induced by the stronger strength have not been entirely cleared. Sometimes a further injection of this dose will clear the symptoms, but occasionally it will be necessary to move to the next weaker solution to clear the symptoms. In these cases it is this 'next weakest' dose that will be considered the neutralizing point. In over 80 per cent of cases the first dose to produce a negative wheal is the neutralizing dose. If a weaker dose than the neutralizing dose is administered, then symptoms will usually recur. This is called under-dosage; the symptoms can be eradicated simply by going back to the next strongest dose, which is obviously the neutralizing level. Thus, in a patient suffering from asthma, wheezing can normally be induced by too strong or too weak a dose, and can be removed by administering the neutralizing dose. Patients find it totally amazing that their asthma can be turned on and off within a few minutes. They find the changes often so impressive that they wish medical sceptics could observe the changes they are experiencing within their own bodies. These changes can also be scientifically validated by monitoring the patient with a peak flow meter.

For inhalant sensitivity we normally start testing on the Number 4 strength (1/625). The reason for this is that some super-sensitive patients may react quite severely to a very strong concentration of inhalant allergen, and secondly the common neutralizing dose for inhaled allergies are the 5, 6 and 7 levels. Obviously we wish to get to the neutralizing level as quickly as possible for each patient and each item. The Number 4 strength intradermally is equivalent, approximately, to a prick test, and so all patients who prick test positive to an inhaled allergen will react to the Number 4 level of the same item when administered intradermally. If the Number 4 level produces a negative result we will go to the Number 3 level; if this is negative, to the Number 2 level and sometimes even to the Number 1 level. Sometimes patients will be distinctly positive, for example, on the Number 2 level, with the production of symptoms, to find that the Number 3 level is negative with the removal of symptoms. Thus these patients are neutralizing on the Number 3 level. These same patients, if they were prick tested for this allergen, would produce only negative results, which explains why prick testing is so unreliable in some patients.

How Neutralization Therapy Works

Currently we know a certain amount about the immunologic process that is involved in the neutralization phenomenon. The fine details, however, are not as yet fully understood and I think it may well be many years before they are. This problem, however, applies to most medical treatments currently available.

- We do not know how painkillers work.
- We do not know how sleeping tablets work.
- We do not know how anti-inflammatory drugs work in relieving the pain and swelling in arthritis.
- We do not know how tranquillizers or anti-depressants work.
- We do not know how conventional incremental desensitization works (or does not work!).

I could go on for a long time in this vein. Most drug treatment has been discovered by chance in a very empirical fashion. New drugs are usually discovered by 'trying out' whole ranges of new synthetic chemicals on animals such as guinea pigs and rats. Those which appear to have the more beneficial effects are then tried on 'higher' animals, such as cats. After animal experimentation the more promising-looking drugs are then tried on human volunteers. The whole process is therefore based much more on trial and error than on any great understanding of the basic mechanism of the disease process being considered.

Neutralization is certainly a very complex immunological phenomenon, about which I give some account in my book, *Arthritis – Allergy, Nutrition and the Environment*. Basically, the immune system is like a million huge armies which have a large variety of weapons and strategies co-ordinated to oppose similarly large armies of allergens, bacteria, viruses, fungi, yeasts and toxins. The homeostatic restoring dose of the offending allergen that is given during a course of neutralization therapy drives the whole system back to its normal balance. Neutralization therapy can level out this tilted balance within a few minutes and turn off the release of histamine and other chemical mediators much more effectively and quickly than any other technique known to humanity.

Administration of Neutralization

After the neutralizing levels for the major inhaled allergens have been determined, they are either administered to the patient by sublingual drops or by subcutaneous injections, which are usually self-administered.

The area under the human tongue (sublingual area) has a good reputation for being an area of high absorbability. Inspection of the area under the tongue will reveal large veins (the sublingual veins). This is, of course, the reason why patients who are taking nitroglycerine tablets to treat angina place these tablets under their tongue, to obtain the most rapid response. Sublingual desensitizing drops are hence placed under the tongue using a special dropper bottle (patients are taught how to do this correctly). The curved dropper bottles produce a carefully calibrated quantity and the solution in the dropper bottles is made up so that each single drop delivered from the pipette contains the precise neutralizing dose of the inhalant to which the patient is sensitive. In other words, one drop delivered from such a bottle can contain neutralizing doses for a number of differing inhaled allergens.

Technicians use a fairly simple mathematical formula to calculate the amount of reagent each patient needs, dependent on the results of the skin testing. Sublingual drops are effective for about five hours, while subcutaneous injections will be effective for two days in most patients. The injections are normally made up in a 0.1 cc dosage; the amount of inhaled allergen in these is of course calculated appropriately.

Of the two methods, my preference is for the subcutaneous injections, although I do use both on my patients. Nowadays, modern insulin syringes are disposable, have a very fine in-built needle, are extremely easy to use and, most important of all, very rarely hurt the patient. Most patients who try both methods of administering their neutralizing doses prefer the injection because it is a little more effective, and the fact that it is only required every two days makes it very convenient.

These desensitizing drops or injections fulfil two purposes. The first is that, within a week or so, they enable the patient to inhale aero-allergens without adverse effect. Secondly, if the desensitization has been administered for a year to one-and-a-half years, the patient becomes desensitized to these inhalants and does not need to take further desensitization treatment.

Disadvantages of Neutralization Therapy

By far the biggest problem with neutralization therapy is the fact that after several weeks or months of this treatment the neutralizing levels can change. Often the specific reason for this change is inexplicable, but in many cases it appears to be a feature of the progressive desensitization that is occurring as treatment continues to be administered. What normally happens is that a patient who has experienced enormous or total relief of asthma suddenly notices that the symptoms are beginning to recur without any obvious change in the environment. In these circumstances re-testing is indicated. Another possible reason for a change in neutralizing levels is the occurrence of a severe attack of flu or a similar viral illness. Whatever the reason for the change, however, re-testing is indicated. Most frequently the re-testing reveals that the neutralizing levels have become stronger. In other words, as the patient has become progressively desensitized, a stronger dose is needed to neutralize his or her symptoms. It is furthermore possible that several months later the neutralization levels will again change to an even stronger level, at which point the levels usually remain stable.

Certainly, instability of neutralizing levels almost inevitably decreases with time.

The main disadvantage with changing neutralizing levels, of course, concerns the inevitable cost to the patient of re-testing and taking time off work for this to be done. If only a few inhalants are involved this is a minor problem, but it can be quite a big problem if multiple allergies are being dealt with. The ongoing cost of the neutralizing injections is comparatively small and this compares favourably with the cost of anti-asthma drugs.

Considering the enormous benefits of this technique these disadvantages are quite small. There is, with the possible exception of enzyme-potentiated desensitization, a technique pioneered by Dr. Len McEwen, no other technique which enables patients to inhale items to which they are sensitive without symptoms. Enzyme-potentiated desensitization has only comparatively few advocates and has been subject to only a small number of clinical trials validating its use. Provocative neutralization therapy has, however, been subjected to many trials (*see Chapter 14*), including one very large one organized by the American ear, nose and throat (ENT) profession, which has established its effectiveness. It is currently used by several thousand physicians in their daily practice, including a high proportion of the ENT specialists in the US.

13

How to Desensitize to Foods and Chemicals

In Chapter 12 the technique of desensitizing people to inhaled allergens by the neutralization technique was described in some detail.

Essentially, the concepts and technique are almost identical when food allergy or chemical sensitivity is involved.

In a patient in whom food sensitivity is a major factor in their asthma, it is of course theoretically possible that the food or foods can be avoided. These food sensitivities may have been discovered during the course of an elimination diet. However, as has been discussed earlier, the most frequent food sensitivities discovered in asthma sufferers are to items such as wheat, corn, cow's milk, yeast, eggs, coffee, soy, cane and beet sugar. These foods have become, during the course of this century, if you like, the building blocks of the Western diet, largely as a result of the processed food industry with all its wonderful concoctions, which many people have become in the habit of relying on totally.

At the end of Chapter 11 there are lists of foods containing wheat, corn, milk, yeast and soy. Any asthma sufferer who has made the discovery that several of these 'building-block foods' are instrumental in his or her asthma will probably be able to avoid them while eating at home. However, attending a wedding reception, a firm's dinner dance, a cocktail party, a business lunch, a dinner party or almost any other social occasion can well become a nightmare.

Accordingly, the vast majority of our patients who are sensitive to major food items request neutralization to enable them to eat the foods to which they are sensitive without recurrence of their asthma.

The Technique of Food Neutralization

Food extracts are obtained from the usual allergy supply companies in the standard 1/10 or 1/20 prick test concentrates. These concentrates contain 50 per cent glycerine, added during the course of the extraction to stabilize the food molecules. This maintains their potency for several years. As with inhaled allergens we use benzyl alcohol in intravenous-quality normal saline to dilute these extracts (serial 1-in-5 dilutions) as described in Chapter 12.

In contrast to inhalant testing, with foods we normally start on the number 1 (1-in-5) or 2 (1-in-25) strengths. As the concentrate contains 50 per cent glycerine, the Number 1 strength (1-in-5) will contain 10 per cent glycerine and the Number 2 strength will contain 2 per cent glycerine. Ten per cent glycerine has a water-attracting (hygroscopic) effect and, as such, will draw fluid into the site of the wheal from the neighbouring tissue. Thus an injection of pure 10 per cent glycerine into the skin will, in most patients, produce a positive wheal reaction. This is *not* because they are sensitive to glycerine, but because of its water-attracting effect. Thus if a Number 1 food skin test is to be judged positive the wheal must grow by more than the 10 per cent glycerine control. In the case of the Number 2 level, as this contains only 2 per cent glycerine this is not enough to have this water-attracting effect.

The most common neutralizing levels for food allergens are the 2, 3 and 4 levels, which contrasts with the 4, 5, 6 and 7 levels in regard to inhalant allergies. It is this single fact which explains, incidentally, why skin prick tests are so totally useless in diagnosing food allergies. Only about one in six food tests will be positive on the Number 4 strength, and it is the number 4 strength which is equivalent to a skin prick test. Dr. Keith Eaton discovered that prick tests in patients with known food allergies had a success rate of only 15 per cent; put another way, this means an 85 per cent failure rate. To emphasize the uselessness of skin prick testing with food allergy, one could make the point that tossing a coin will give a 50 per cent reliability and so skin prick testing is three times worse than the tossing of a coin. Countless patients, in my experience, have been told that they are not sensitive to a food on the basis of a negative prick test, even when they have been convinced from their own observations that a specific food upsets them.

The single most common neutralizing level is the Number 2 level, with the Number 3 level being the next most common. Rarely, patients may even neutralize on a Number 1 level. In these circumstances they may develop symptoms on a negative Number 2 test (indicating under-dosage), which then become relieved by giving the stronger dose, the Number 1 level. This then proves that the Number 1 is the neutralizing dose.

Diagnosis of Food Allergy by Skin Test

Most patients with food allergy are sorted out by an elimination diet; the skin testing in these patients is used only to determine their neutralizing levels to foods which have been already identified, but which need neutralization.

An extension of the skin test technique is to use it for diagnosis. Clearly, if positive wheal reactions and symptoms can be obtained in the course of skin testing there is no absolute need to go through an elimination dietary procedure. Furthermore, whereas an elimination diet can take five or six weeks, during which time major social occasions may need to be avoided, a comprehensive skin testing programme can be completed in about 2½ to 3 days of intensive testing. A workable procedure involves scanning about 34 major foods with intradermal provocative skin tests. The reaction to all 34 foods is tested, and neutralizing doses are obtained for all those items to which there is a positive reaction. At the end of the test programme, the patient is only allowed to eat those foods tested and to take neutralizing injections to cover all those items to which a sensitivity has been found. The advantages of this approach are considerable.

- The test programme is completed in a few days.
- The patient does not need to assess his or her own response.
- There is no need to abandon drugs, which in the case of the severe asthmatic might be hazardous.
- If the patient lives a long way from the clinic the test procedure saves a whole series of long journeys at various stages of the elimination diet.
- If multiple food sensitivities are involved, these tests will be inevitable anyway, even after the elimination diet, because it will be necessary to desensitize the patient to a large number of foods.
- In some patients their reactions to foods are very insidious and can be picked up better by skin test.
- In most cases the treatment programme is very successful.

The disadvantages of this treatment, as opposed to the elimination diet followed by desensitization to specifically identified food allergens, are:

- The skin test technique picks up adapted food allergies as well as non-adapted food allergies (*see Chapter 15*). Hence the number of foods to which someone reacts often appears more complicated than it really is, and a degree of overtreatment is almost certainly inevitable using this technique.

- Patients do not know whether they are going to see a successful outcome until after the treatment is completed, whereas after the first stage of the elimination diet most discover for themselves that, once removed from their major food allergies, they feel much better.

- Going through an elimination diet probably gives the patient a better idea than skin testing as to which food allergens cause severe reactions and which mild, and also the patient may learn to associate certain symptoms with certain foods.

- The elimination diet is an educative programme, whereas skin testing is far less so in itself. Consequently, at the end of a skin testing programme the patient must learn to use only those items which have been evaluated. This involves some education into the way in which multiple foods are made up and what they contain. For example, at the end of the testing programme it is probable that wholemeal bread will be permitted, but not white bread because the chemicals (bleaching agents, anti-staling agents, etc.) added to this have not been assessed. Thus, at the end of such a programme a patient could conceivably sabotage all the careful work that has been done up to that point by, for example, eating white bread. If the patient is sensitive to the chemicals in white bread and is not covered for them by desensitizing drops or injections, this may in itself be enough to cause symptoms to continue. This is just one example; I could give many others.

After remaining on the foods tested for a few weeks and presumably observing a huge improvement in their asthma, patients can then extend their repertoire of foods by bringing back into the diet one single food at a time and observing any response.

Chemical Desensitization

With biological inhalant neutralization and with food neutralization, the effect at first is to protect the patient, but eventually after a period of time, usually 1½ to 3 years, the patient is completely desensitized and is able to eat or inhale former allergens with impunity. In the case of chemicals there is no doubt that the usual protection can be afforded, but long-term desensitization is more doubtful. Some physicians in the

US refer to chemical neutralization as 'cheater drops' rather than desensitization, as they feel the neutralization is just 'cheating the symptoms'. Having said this, I have certainly had some patients who claim very definitely that they have been desensitized to chemicals by this technique. However, I usually regard chemical neutralization as a short-term expedient, while long term we attack the nutritional basis of patients' malfunctioning detoxification system (*see Chapter 7*) and reduce their exposure to the continuously inhaled chemicals.

Skin testing with chemicals is particularly important diagnostically and if, for example, gas or formaldehyde sensitivity is discovered, the possibility of eradicating these contacts may be worth exploring as discussed in Chapter 7.

The most common chemicals that we test are:

1. natural gas
2. synthetic ethanol
3. formaldehyde
4. petrol
5. diesel
6. cigarette smoke
7. cigar smoke
8. pipe smoke
9. perfumes
10. phenol (the gas that comes off soft plastics)
11. toluene (from gloss paint).

Synthetic ethanol is the core hydrocarbon present in natural gas. We start testing on the Number 1 solution (the 1-in-5 dilution of the concentrate we obtain from allergy supply companies). Having discovered the neutralizing concentrations in the ways described earlier in this chapter, we administer chemical neutralization by sublingual drops, as we do not consider that patients should regularly give themselves injections of chemicals, however dilute.

The sublingual neutralizing drops, however, only work for three or four hours, but can be very useful in, for example, protecting a patient from traffic fumes during car journeys. They can also be very useful in protecting patients against cigarette, cigar or pipe smoke on a visit to friends or out to a restaurant or pub.

With regard to perfumes, we have cheap and expensive perfume extracts on our testing shelves. Considering the complexity of the various chemicals that go into the average perfume, it always surprises me that these crude mixtures work as well as they do; many patients have been able to avoid asthma attacks at social gatherings by the use of these drops.

Hence, sublingual neutralizing drops work quite well against occasionally encountered chemical sensitivities, but they are much less helpful when the patient is continuously exposed to a chemical such as gas or formaldehyde from carpets, fabrics and chipboard. Gas levels are present in houses fairly continuously and are not related only to those times when, for example, a gas cooker is on. The levels stay high in a house for several days after all utilities are completely turned off. Thus, when a patient feels greatly improved when gas utilities are turned off temporarily, the only real solution is to move the boiler to a shed outside the house and replace the cooker with an electric one.

Similarly, major sources of formaldehyde, such as carpets, can be removed temporarily; if an obvious benefit accrues, the removal perhaps should become permanent and an alternative floor covering substituted.

Clinical Trials of Desensitization by Neutralization

It must have become obvious to the reader by now that the success of neutralization treatment is pretty vital to this whole approach. As such, it behoves me to set out the clinical evidence which has accumulated so far that supports the efficacy of this technique. There have, in fact, been a large number of clinical trials carried out in the US, and four in the UK, of which three were on human beings and one on horses. These trials involved patients with a variety of symptoms that appeared to be related to food or inhalant allergies. They include asthma, migraine, colitis, and rhinitis. Although some of these trials, therefore, do not concentrate on asthma, I think it is reasonable to assume that, if the adverse effects of a food or inhaled allergen can be neutralized, it does not really matter which symptoms the food or inhaled allergen is causing. Certainly, this is the common experience of physicians working in this field.

'Horse Trials'

One of the four British trials[1] was carried out by my own clinic and sprang from work that we had been asked to do with horses. Asthma is a big problem in horses, where it is called either Heaves, or chronic obstructive pulmonary disease (COPD for short). This condition can completely wreck the career of top-flight race horses, as drug medications are specifically not allowed before racing. We have had the immense satisfaction of seeing many horses restored to competitive racing or jumping. We soon realized that a successful outcome to a study involving horses would add considerable weight to those studies performed with human beings, as it is difficult to imagine any sort of placebo effect occurring in a horse. It is always difficult for a private clinic, such as my own, to organize a placebo-controlled trial, as patients do not pay good money to be given placebo treatment.

In this study, 14 out of 18 horses (78 per cent) showed at least a 75 per cent reduction in their asthma symptomatology.

It is of interest to note that the three COPD cases which did not respond to treatment had all had ongoing symptoms for significantly longer than the mean duration, and in one case the onset of cardiac failure clearly affected the result. Also of interest was the fact that the onset of improvement in symptoms in these horses was rather slower than we normally see in human beings.

Disease	Number of Cases	Number Improved	Onset of <2 Weeks	Improvement 2–6 Weeks	Symptoms >6 Weeks
COPD	18	15 (83%)	4	6	5

Another part of this study concerned urticaria, where 11 out of the 12 cases improved (92 per cent).

Disease	Number of Cases	Number Improved	Onset of <2 Weeks	Improvement 2–6 Weeks	Symptoms >6 Weeks
Urticaria	12	11 (92%)	6	3	2

These results with urticaria represent a staggeringly high success rate, as this condition is regarded by most veterinary surgeons and dermatologists (human) as incurable.

The two other conditions we looked at were headshaking and sweet itch. Vets consider that headshaking has many causes, of which allergy may be one, and this is probably reflected in the fact that we only obtained a 38 per cent success rate in this condition. In the horses with sweet itch, two out of three improved, both within two weeks.

A wide range of allergens were used in the inhalant tests. The inhaled substances included housedust, house dust mite, pollens, and hay and straw dust. Mould allergens used were extracted from 46 different species. Extracts of food included wheat, corn, oats, barley, soya, beet sugar and can sugar. A *Culicoides* sp. allergen was used for three horses suffering from sweet itch.

Intradermal Testing and Neutralization

To return to human beings, the first clinical trial to demonstrate the validity of neutralization therapy was organized by Dr. Joseph Miller of Mobile, Alabama.[2] Dr. Miller was, as described earlier, the physician most connected with clarifying, organizing and teaching others about this concept in the first place.

Patients who were selected for this study had illnesses strongly suspected to be caused by food sensitivity. Each of them was extensively tested for all the commonly-eaten foods by intradermal provocative neutralization testing. The neutralizing doses of the implicated foods were combined into a single injection solution specifically for each individual. The injections were self-administered subcutaneously daily for 20 days. Patients were restricted to eating those foods that had been assessed.

Placebo injections were prepared which were indistinguishable from the injections containing the active neutralizing doses. The placebo injections were also self-administered daily for 20 days. The first series of injections to be used (active or placebo) was decided randomly by the toss of a coin by a third party. Thus, neither the patient nor the physician was aware of which extracts were used. This trial therefore qualifies for the title of a double-blind trial. In the summary it was stated that the superiority of active extract over placebo extract for the eight patients involved was clearly significant, at a 99.8 per cent level of confidence. In most patients the active extract was rapidly and markedly effective and the placebo was totally ineffective.

Case No. 1, for example, was a 29-year-old with severe migraine problems recurrent since early childhood, becoming progressively worse. In the preceding six months the headaches had awoken her in the early morning every day. She reported that headaches followed the ingestion of coffee, chocolate, beef, pork and ice cream, amongst other things. She had been taking potent drugs by mouth and potent injections for nine years. Additional symptoms included recurrent vertigo, buzzing in the ears (tinnitus), nausea, abdominal cramps and depression.

The first series of injections administered was of active extract. After the third injection she required no further medication and was completely free of headache, vertigo, tinnitus and depression for the remainder of the 20 days. She stated that this was the longest period she had ever gone without a headache in her entire life. The nausea and abdominal cramps were present very mildly.

During the second series of injections (placebo) the headaches and all her other symptoms returned on the fourth day and remained severe for the rest of the 20-day period. On the third series of injections (active) her symptoms had almost cleared by the third day and she remained virtually symptom-free for the rest of the 20-day period. On the fourth series (placebo) her symptoms returned again, but not as severely as on the second series. This is a common finding in this type of trial. By the time the second placebo phase has started, the patient has had 40 desensitizing injections during the two active phases and the patient is beginning to become desensitized. This desensitizing effect carries over into the placebo phase, despite discontinuation of the active injections, and provides some carry-over protection. Although this is evidence that a long-term desensitization effect occurs, it tends to diminish the difference between the active and placebo phases and thus understates the advantage of the active extract.

Another case in this study was also a severe migraine sufferer. She had had severe migraine accompanied by nausea and vomiting since early childhood, which had become progressively worse in the seven months prior to the study. She had been awakened by severe headaches every morning at 4 o'clock. She had very frequent injections of narcotics such as pethidine in high dosage. Every three weeks or so these injections failed her and she was hospitalized and heavily sedated for three to seven days. She herself did not think it was likely that foods were related to her migraine.

The first series of injections (placebo) did not beneficially affect her at all. In the second series (active) the headaches became noticeably less severe after the third injection. Her photophobia and acne also became markedly better. Only a few mild headaches and one migraine occurred in the 20-day evaluation period. On the third series (placebo) she went rapidly downhill and by the sixth day her pethidine was no longer able to control her symptoms and she was readmitted to hospital for five days. The headaches continued in their original severity and frequency for the rest of the 20-day period. On the fourth series (active) she noticed improvement again on the fifth day and had no severe headaches for the rest of this phase.

In April 1984 Dr. William J. Rea and his colleagues at the Environmental Health Centre in Dallas[3] reported on a similar trial in their paper entitled 'Elimination of Oral Food Challenge Reactions by Ingestion of Food Extracts'. This trial was, in my opinion, attempting to do something rather more difficult than that which had been demonstrated in Dr. Miller's trial. Dr. Rea was attempting to turn off deliberately-induced food-allergic reactions with a single neutralizing dose of the food. As demonstrated in Dr. Miller's trial, several sequential daily injections are often required before maximum benefit is obtained. I know this also from my own experience.

In their summary of the trial, the authors wrote that the results of this study were consistent with previous double-blind studies in providing support for the existence of the neutralizing dose effect that is different from and superior to the effect of the placebo. The responses in terms of signs and symptoms were divided into six possible variables. For each of these six variables a very significant difference was found between the neutralization and placebo situations. This demonstrated the effectiveness of the neutralizing dose in providing relief of symptomatology. The return of oral food challenge reactions when the placebo injections were used further emphasized the validity of the neutralizing dose method. Extremely elaborate precautions were taken to make these tests absolutely foolproof in terms of the double-blind, etc. and full details of this are given in the original paper. The paper concluded with the statement, 'It appears that the phenomenon of subcutaneous food neutralization can be scientifically endorsed for clinical use in the treatment of food reactions.'

Hyperactivity in Children

Another study of neutralizing therapy was published in the *Journal of Learning Disabilities* in April 1984.[4] The purpose of this study was to determine by double-blind study whether the hyperkinetic syndrome (better known in Britain as hyperactivity) in children was at least partly because of individual reactions to foods, dyes, and inhalants. After being assessed by intradermal and sublingual testing, each patient was provided with composite individual extracts. As in Dr. Miller's trial, an active phase and a placebo phase were employed. Each child's behaviour in each phase was monitored by parents, teachers and a psychologist. Significant improvement was noticed in 11 out of the 14 children when treated with the active preparations, as opposed to the placebo.

Inhaled Allergy

In the field of inhaled allergy problems there are as yet only four published trials relating to neutralization therapy. The first, by Dr. Schiff *et al.*, was published in *The Journal of Allergy and Clinical Immunology* in 1983.[5] This trial was carried out entirely in the laboratory.

The effect of neutralizing therapy on patients who had asthma induced by reaction to animal furs was evaluated using peak flow meters and other similar instruments.

All patients were first challenged with increasing amounts of animal dander until the amount required to cause a 20 per cent decrease in the peak flow was determined. Neutralizing levels were then obtained in the traditional way to the specific animal danders that were being used. The patients were given either no treatment, placebo treatment or active neutralization treatment. The results showed that the FEB1 (force expiratory volume in one second) decreased by 27.7 per cent from baseline in the controls, 25.9 per cent after placebo injections, but by only 9.4 per cent after the active neutralizing injections. They concluded that there was a distinct diminution of animal dander-induced bronchospasm with neutralization therapy, which may well have important therapeutic implications.

These results are particularly good when it is considered that this improvement resulted from a single injection. As the previously quoted trials have demonstrated, there is a build-up effect after several injections have been given.

Another trial, published in *Clinical Allergy* in 1986,[6] was carried out at the Middlesex Hospital in London by Dr. Jonathan Brostoff and Dr. Glenis Scadding of the Department of Immunology. They entitled the trial 'Low Dose Sublingual Therapy in Patients with Allergic Rhinitis due to House Dust Mite'. By low-dose therapy they meant neutralization therapy. Summarizing their results, they stated that in a double-blind placebo-controlled cross-over trial, low-dose sublingual therapy with housedust mite was effective in relieving symptoms in 72 per cent of the group of patients with perennial rhinitis caused by housedust mite ($P<0.03$). Following active treatment, there was a significant increase in morning peak nasal inspiratory flow rate ($P<0.01$) in those who improved (13 out of 18) and resistance to nasal provocation with housedust mite also increased, in some cases up to 1,000-fold ($P<0/05$). The potential for oral desensitization is great, and further studies on this form of treatment are needed.

Interestingly, if we analyse these results we see that 13 out of 18 patients preferred the active preparation (the specific neutralizing dose), as their overall symptoms were improved by this treatment. However, four preferred the placebo (not because it provided any benefit, but because their symptoms were made worse by the active treatment). This would seem to mean that, in four patients, the neutralizing level on first assessment was incorrect. Re-testing will normally convert this situation into one of benefit. Only one patient was undecided and so was probably a genuine failure. Most patients in my experience have an even better response with neutralization for housedust mite administered by subcutaneous injection.

Recently, a further study, again involving Dr. Jonathan Brostoff but having as its main author Dr. Michael Radcliffe, has emanated from the Department of Immunology at University College London Hospital. The paper was entitled 'Allergen-specific Low-dose Immunotherapy in Perennial Allergic Rhinitis, A Double-blind, Placebo-controlled Cross-over Study'.[7] The summary stated that in a double-blind, placebo-controlled cross-over study, 36 adults with perennial allergic rhinitis were treated with daily subcutaneous injections of inhaled allergens, the doses of which had been predetermined by intradermal testing. The dose chosen for each allergen was the maximum intradermally tolerated dose of that allergen, which is the standard definition of the neutralizing dose. Of the 27 who expressed a preference, 78 per cent preferred the active preparation and 22 per cent the placebo. Significant symptom relief was apparent on an analysis of total rhinitis symptom scores ($P=0.006$), nasal blockage ($P=0.02$), nasal discharge ($P=0.06$), post-nasal drip ($P=0.02$) and anosmia (loss of smell) ($P=0.02$). These results support the validity of allergen-specific low-dose immunotherapy (neutralization).

A further British trial was carried out at the Royal Liverpool Hospital under the guidance of my long-term friend and colleague, Dr. Ronald Finn, who is a Consultant Physician at that hospital and an ex-President of the British Society for Allergy and Environmental Medicine. The trial was published in 1988[8] and involved treatment programmes for both inhalant and food allergens.

To summarize the trial, it can be said that 53 patients with a variety of conditions were placed on a treatment programme comprising neutralization therapy plus selected environmental control. Overall there was a success rate of 66 per cent in a group of patients who had long-standing intractable disease. Most of the patients were secondary or tertiary referrals and had had so much medical attention that placebo effects were unlikely. Those patients who were highly allergic had a higher success rate (87 per cent) than the others, where the success rate was 44 per cent. Patients were considered highly allergic if their neutralizing levels were as low as Number 5. Patients with specific conditions, such as eczema, asthma and urticaria ($P > 0.05$), did better than other patients.

The authors concluded with the observation that these results are incompatible with a placebo effect or with a natural remission of the disease, and indicate that the overall success rate resulted from a genuine effect of the treatment regime.

Sublingual Provocation Trials

There have been several reports relating to the efficacy and validity of sublingual testing for food allergies. These trials have not concerned themselves with the neutralization aspect, but have concentrated on whether patients can distinguish between a placebo and a sublingually-administered extract of a food to which they are sensitive. My view is that sublingual testing is markedly inferior to intradermal testing, as it relies entirely on the patient's subjective response both for diagnosis and for determination of the neutralizing level. The intradermal test has the wheal appearance, indicating positivity or negativity, which is extremely helpful because, of course, it is independent of the patient's subjective feelings. Furthermore, I have the impression clinically that some foods are not absorbed well under the tongue and that this is a potent cause of inaccuracy.

In 1981 *The Journal of Biological Psychiatry*[9] published a paper by Dr. D. King entitled 'Can Allergic Exposure Provoke Psychological Symptoms? A Double-blind Test'. This trial evaluated allergy patients who had at least one psychological symptom, such as anxiety, depression, confusion, or a problem with concentration. The question to be determined was, 'Did sublingual provocation with a specific food induce psychological symptoms more frequently than a placebo?' and 30 patients were challenged with selected foods and with triple-distilled water as a placebo. The trial was subdivided into four types: (1) allergen trials — four allergy-producing foods, each given three times; (2) placebo trials — two tests, each given three times; (3) base rate trials in which the subjects received nothing sublingually but nevertheless received a complete evaluation; (4) open placebo trials to assess any biological reactivity of the placebo (three trials). Great care was taken to ensure that the test was properly double-blind, including the evaluation. Average symptom scores for psychological symptoms were four times higher after allergy-producing foods than after placebo provocation.

The difference was highly statistically significant (P=0.001). Therefore, Dr. King would appear to have demonstrated that challenge sublingually with foods known to produce allergy can produce psychological symptoms much more frequently than placebo.

In contrast, there have been two studies which have been published and do not confirm the results of all these other studies. The studies were by C. Lehman and Dr. D.L. Jewett.[10] Both of these studies were done, in my view, very badly, and the authors clearly didn't understand many of the fundamental premises of this type of testing. Allergists, who are highly experienced in intradermal neutralization testing, have pulled these two studies apart. The Jewett study was in fact originally turned down by several allergy journals on these grounds, but eventually surfaced many years later in the prestigious *New England Journal of Medicine*, where it caused a major furore in the allergy establishment. The motive for publishing this in such an establishment journal is not difficult to fathom in my opinion. An account of these studies can be found in my book, *Arthritis – Allergy, Nutrition and the Environment*.

In total contrast to these last two papers, in September 1988 the American Academy of Otolaryngology (called ENT specialists in the UK) published a study, which it had sponsored, in the *Journal of Otolaryngology*.[11] The paper was entitled 'Provocation Neutralization – A 2-Part Study. Part I – The intracutaneous provocative food test. A multi-centre comparison study'. This study investigated the reliability of the intradermal provocative neutralization test as a diagnostic tool for food sensitivity. Thirty-seven patients were tested for five identical food allergens by eight physicians in different geographical locations in the US.

All the testing started on the Number 1 strength of each food (a 1-in-5 solution of the concentrate), and both skin reactions and symptom response were noted. These completely double-blind skin tests were performed on patients known to have certain food sensitivities as determined earlier by oral challenge food tests. The authors emphasized the importance of having the food in the diet when the skin tests were performed, as the test is more reliable in these circumstances. The study showed that the provocation of symptoms was 75 per cent efficient when compared to the oral food challenge test. The provocation of food symptoms had a specificity of 92 per cent, but was only 60 per cent sensitive. In other words, if symptoms were induced on the skin test you could be very sure that the patient was sensitive to that food, but symptoms would not occur on some foods on skin test, despite the fact that the patient had earlier reacted to that food on oral challenge.

The production of positive skin readings was 77 per cent efficient, with a more balanced 72 per cent specificity and 80 per cent sensitivity. Thus, the use of the skin wheal reaction, by itself, will miss fewer guilty foods, but falsely implicate more innocent foods. Falsely implicating a few innocent foods is not really a major problem, as they will do no harm added to the patient's neutralizing vaccine. These reactions probably represent potential (adapted) food sensitivities in any case, and will probably help the patient in the long term.

Thus the combination of observing symptom responses and wheal responses will miss few positive skin reactions, and makes this test demonstrably second only to the elimination diet in terms of reliability.

The second part of this study was labelled 'Subcutaneous Neutralization Therapy – A Multi-Centre Study'.[12] Seven of the original eight physicians who participated in the first study were involved, and a total of 33 patients were evaluated.

This was a *triple-blind cross-over study*. Each patient underwent three two-week treatment sessions, rather like the Miller study discussed at the beginning of this chapter. A placebo injection was used in one of these treatment sessions, and the active vaccine was used in the other two. Injections were self-administered daily in all three treatment sessions, and there was a week off in between each treatment session. The number of foods treated per patient was between one and 13, the majority being treated with three to five foods. Great care was taken to ensure that the patients could not tell in any way between the treatment injections and the placebo injection. The patients' diet did not alter at all throughout the whole procedure.

Improvement, compared with the placebo injections, was reported by 65 per cent of the patients, and a worsening by 23 per cent. No difference was reported by 12 per cent. Aggravation of symptoms by neutralization indicates accurate diagnosis but provision of the wrong treatment dose. In the usual clinical settings these individuals are recognized and re-tested for a shift in their neutralizing levels, or some technical inaccuracy, and their dose is altered. (I don't think their nurses were as good as mine!) Such action normally reverses the negative treatment response to distinctly positive. This indicates that overall provocation neutralization in a clinical setting should be beneficial at least 75 per cent of the time, and this would be enhanced by supplementary dietary manipulation.

When results of treatment are reported to be no better than placebo, this would indicate one of three possibilities:

1. The symptoms were not caused by food allergy.
2. The symptoms were caused by an allergy for which the patient was not tested.
3. The symptoms were caused by a food allergy for which the patient was treated but obtained no relief.

Considering the number of things that could go wrong when approaching the problem solely by this method, I think that the figure of 75 per cent is very good, and certainly better than any other 'quick-fix' non-elimination diet procedure.

The results so impressed the American Academy of Otolaryngic Allergy (especially when combined with the other trials described earlier in this chapter) that they recommended that intradermal skin testing, followed by neutralization therapy, was the treatment of choice for allergic conditions such as rhinitis and other related illnesses. As the various manifestations of rhinitis are the largest single problem that ENT specialists encounter, over half the ENT specialists in the US currently use this technique. As there are over 4,000 ENT specialists, this has enormously increased the number of physicians worldwide using this technique. I have talked informally to a number of these ENT consultants, and they were uniformly enthusiastic about its use, especially in rhinitis, which is a condition that has been hitherto very difficult to help. As one of them succinctly said to me: 'Neutralization is the only thing that is worth a damn!'

As neutralization therapy is now supported as the 'treatment of choice' by the American Academy of Environmental Medicine, The Academy of Otolaryngic Allergy, and The Pan American Allergy Association, a conservative estimate is that 3,000 physicians in the US alone use this technique. There are many others in Canada, Australia, New Zealand and the UK.

15

The Roots of Allergy

Why then do some people develop sensitivities to dust, dust mites, moulds, pollens, animals, chemicals and food, and others do not?

Genetic susceptibility clearly plays a part but, as this book has demonstrated, an environmental trigger is required as well. Thus, the whole thing can perhaps be summarized by the equation, Genetic Susceptibility × Environmental Trigger. We have already touched on the probable reasons for the development of inhaled allergy and chemical sensitivity, and to recap on these we should again mention the phenomenon of tolerance induction. The prime function of our immune system (defence army) is to distinguish invaders which may be harmful from those which may be harmless. Thus, the immune system should act decisively against disease-causing microbes, but not against 'harmless' items like dust mites, pollens and foods. The act of learning to distinguish and shrug off items that are harmless is termed *tolerance induction*. The role of chemical sensitivity in this respect is dealt with extensively in Chapter 7. The base causes of this problem would appear to be high exposure to chemicals occurring at the same time as a diminution in the intake of certain trace minerals, B vitamins and amino acids.

In Chapter 9 we have explored the role of deficiencies of magnesium, vitamin B_{12}, B_6 and vitamin C in causing asthma.

Food sensitivity may lead to a type of gastric inflammation which reduces the acidity in the stomach (achlorhydria), which then leads to a reduction of intrinsic factor release and subsequent vitamin B_{12} deficiency. This deficiency can be remedied by injections of vitamin B_{12}. The effect that a combination of nutritional factors can have on animals (and by implication, humans) was brilliantly demonstrated in 1945 in what has become known as the Pottenger Cat Studies.

The Pottenger Cat Studies

Drug companies are well aware that in most respects cats respond similarly to human beings, and so they are widely used for testing drugs. These experiments were suggested by Pottenger's observation that cats fed on a raw meat and untreated milk diet were much better operative risks than those fed cooked meat and untreated milk. In a series of experiments, one group of cats was fed on a diet of two-thirds raw meat, one-third milk and cod-liver oil. A second group was fed on a diet of two-thirds cooked meat, one-third milk and cod-liver oil. Nine hundred cats were studied over a period of 10 years.

The cats receiving raw meat reproduced normally, had few abortions, nursed their young well, had very good behaviour patterns and a high resistance to infections and parasites.

The cats receiving the cooked meat reproduced poorly in general and there was an abortion rate of 25 per cent in the first generation, increasing to 70 per cent in the second generation. Many cats died in labour and the mortality rate in the kittens was high. The cats were irritable and difficult to handle, and skin lesions and allergies were frequent and became progressively worse from generation to generation while the cats remained on the same diet. In addition, the oral arches narrowed, and osteomyelitis, cardiac lesions, thyroid disease, nephritis, hepatitis, arthritis, asthma and many other conditions familiar to human beings all became common. Of the cats maintained entirely on the cooked meat and milk diet, the kittens of the third generation were so degenerated that none of them survived the first six months of life, thereby terminating the strain.

Cats of the first and second generation cooked meat group were later returned to a raw meat diet. Of enormous significance was the fact that it took three to four generations before the offspring regained good health. At the beginning of this century people in the Western world started to eat highly refined and processed foods, with a high percentage of our food cooked. We are, therefore, in approximately the third or fourth generation of eating such foods, and increasingly we are getting the same diseases that the Pottenger cats did.

There follows from this work the enormous implication that a condition which may be currently considered genetic in origin could stem from poor nutrition in an earlier generation. The other, less happy implication is that really adequate nutrition may fail to correct chronic diseases within one generation. This is not to say, however, that allergy management and meganutrition could not do the same job.

This trial report is not a plea for human beings to exist on raw food and milk! It is, however, a demonstration that inadequate nutrition can have a disastrous effect in terms of disease on one species, and there is no reason to believe that inadequate diet could not have the same effect on human beings. Pottenger surmised that the problem could well be the denaturing of protein by heat. Certainly, heating meat alters its physio-chemical state in the same way as processing other foods will alter their ability to remain perfect for the maintenance of health.

A Monotonous, Repetitive Diet

Humans have eaten vegetables, fruit, fish and meat since the Stone Age. Physicians working with food-allergic patients know that these foods, especially in their organic form, are for most patients the safest. The reason for this probably is that we have, as a species, eaten these foods for two to three million years and we are hence fairly well adapted to them. Any of our forebears who could not tolerate these types of food have probably tended to die out. The Stone Age diet was conceived by Dr. Richard Mackarness as a relatively safe diet on which many food-allergic patients would improve, as it avoids all the common food allergens. A perusal of the food trials shows wheat to be the most common item implicated with asthma. Corn, milk, eggs, cane and beet sugar, yeast and soya beans are also amongst the more common offenders.

Although bread is regarded by many people to be the 'staff of life', most people are surprised to learn that cereals such as wheat and corn are a relatively recent addition to the human diet. Corn was originally planted in Egypt 4,000 years ago, but there is no evidence of cereals being grown in Britain prior to the Roman invasion around 2,000 years ago. Yeast has probably been used for about 8,000 years, originally to make scrumpy. Sugar was unknown in Britain until cane sugar was brought from the West Indies in the 16th century, only about 400 years ago.

Soya beans have been introduced into Britain only since 1955. They now crop up in a multitude of ways, usually in the form of soya-bean oil or soya-bean flour. Soya-bean oil is found in many wholemeal breads. It is also present, usually vaguely labelled as vegetable oil, in margarines, ice cream, salad dressings and mayonnaise. Soya-bean flour is also found in sausages, luncheon meats and confectionery. Thus, most of our major foods have only been in our diet for a couple of hundred – or thousand – years and, in terms of evolution and adaptation, two thousand years is only yesterday.

In Chapter 11 I detailed the multitude of ways in which corn creeps into most people's everyday diet. Many people eat corn in over 10 different ways every day of their lives. The invention of complex food mixtures by the food industry has made it very easy to eat small amounts of wheat, corn, milk, eggs, soy, cane and beet sugar very frequently throughout the day. It would appear that this frequent 'peppering' of our enzyme systems by these foods is very important in the engendering of food sensitivity.

Part of the evidence for this is that it very frequently turns out that foods which people eat most often and most addictively are the ones to which they are sensitive. Admittedly, by the time an individual is seen by the doctor, the addictive factor may be due to the allergy having developed.

Further evidence is provided by observations related to the development of tolerance to foods that at one time produced allergy. If an allergic food is left out of the diet for a period of between three months and two years, tolerance will develop in most instances. It is then observed that, if the food is only eaten about once every four or five days, this tolerance will be maintained. If the food is eaten more frequently, the tolerance is usually destroyed and an allergic response will again result. These observations are the basis of the rotation diet, which is often useful in the management of food allergies. The idea of such a diet is that no food is repeated more than once every four or five days. On such a diet new food allergies virtually never occur, but it is of course difficult to maintain socially. Nevertheless, the effectiveness of such regimes is further proof that the frequency with which a food is ingested is very important in the causation of allergy.

Candida Hypersensitivity

This subject has already been discussed in Chapter 8. Here it is only described in the context in which it may dovetail with other basic causes of allergy. A few years ago, an article in *The Lancet* covered a controlled study indicating that patients with food or skin allergies had leaky mucous membranes which could admit many more protein molecules than was normal. Patients thus developed multiple food and chemical sensitivities because antibodies were formed to the antigenic proteins in food, pollens, and even their own microbiological flora of the gut. This flora includes fungi, such as Candida, trichophyton and epidermophyton. Mucous membranes can also be made to leak by excessive exposure to toxic chemicals, and almost certainly by nutritional deficiencies. The critical mechanisms underlying the food sensitivity problem are, like those underlying the chemical sensitivity problem, almost certainly related to nutritional deficiencies, but in the case of food sensitivity the whole mechanism is not worked out in the detail that we see with chemical sensitivity and the P450 cytochrome system described in great detail in Chapter 7. However, food sensitivity is almost certainly linked to leaky mucosal membranes in the intestine, which certainly in part can be caused by zinc deficiency, as well as achlorhydria. My opinion, based on general experience of dealing with patients rather than hard clinical data, is that the Candida hypersensitivity problem is also probably quite important in some cases of asthma. In many patients these factors interweave to produce the final result. Quite probably, once the situation occurs in which the development of food sensitivity is likely, repeated ingestion of a certain food that is new to our diet will then make it more likely that an allergy will develop.

Resistance and Adaptation

Up to now I have dwelt almost exclusively on the various factors that constitute the insult to the host, that is, the individual. As with all equations, however, the final result depends on the interplay of two factors: (1) the nature of the insult or attack on the host; (2) the resistance and natural adaptive resources of the host.

The work that has most clarified this was done by Hans Selye, the eminent physiologist, working in his laboratory at the University of Montreal. Selye's work on what is termed 'the general adaptation syndrome' will almost certainly eventually rank among the greatest medical discoveries of all time; he has clarified the mechanisms of adaptation to stress. This does not just mean psychological stress but also and more importantly the struggle of the human body to stay healthy in the face of the whole gamut of potentially harmful agents with which it is in daily contact. Selye has defined stress as the rate at which wear and tear is induced in the body by the whole process of living.

It is now known that cortisone, which is produced by the cortex of our adrenal glands, is our main defence against allergic reactions of all types. Selye was the first to demonstrate that cortisone has a protective effect and is also able to mobilize the body's other defences against allergic reactions and other harmful events. In 1946 Selye published a letter in the journal *Nature* entitled, 'A Syndrome Produced by Diverse Nocuous Agents'. The letter starts as follows:

> Experiments on rats show that, if the organism is severely damaged by acute, non-specific noxious agents, such as exposure to cold, surgical injury, excessive muscular exercise or intoxications with sublethal doses of diverse drugs, a typical syndrome appears, the symptoms of which are independent of the nature of the damaging agent or the pharmacological type of drug employed and represent rather a response to damage as such.

Later in the letter Selye describes the three stages of the general adaptation syndrome. Stage 1 (the alarm reaction) starts about 6 to 48 hours after the initial injury. It is akin to what most doctors refer to as surgical shock and is characterized by low blood pressure, loss of muscle tone and shrinkage of the adrenal glands as they pump out as much cortisone as possible. There are also other symptoms, such as leakage of fluid from the smaller blood vessels into the surrounding tissues.

Stage 2 starts about 48 hours after the original injury. There is now considerable enlargement of the adrenal glands; the swelling in the tissues, produced by the leakage of fluid from the blood vessels, starts to subside. The pituitary gland, which controls virtually all the other glands in the body, produces increased amounts of a hormone (adreno-cortico-stimulating hormone) which in turn causes the adrenal glands to produce more cortisone.

When further small repeated doses of the harmful stimulus are given, be it an allergy-producing stimulus or any other, resistance is built up. Hence the órganism adapts and, in this phase, no outward symptoms appear.

In Selye's experiments, if the rats were removed at this stage from the harmful stress, for example the persistent cold stimulus, they would lose their newly-acquired resistance to the cold within a few days. When reintroduced to the cold environment they would have to go through the Stage 1 alarm reaction. Conversely, if the rats were left in the cold, they continued adapting for a long time, apparently having grown completely used to it.

This is what has been described in Chapter 6 of this book, in the section on masking to foods. This mechanism of masking represents the continued application of the harmful stimulus and the body's adapted response to it. The exaggerated adverse response (Rinkel's hyperacute response), when the body is re-exposed to a given food after a period (five days plus) of avoiding it, is a Stage 1 alarm reaction.

If the rats continued to be exposed for a long time to the cold stimulus, they seemed at first to be perfectly well. After a period of time, however, they became ill and eventually died. They had entered a stage of maladaption, and eventually a stage of exhaustion. The symptoms in this Stage 3 (maladaption and then exhaustion) were similar to those of Stage 1 (the alarm stage). In Stage 3, only complete removal of the harmful stimulus would produce a healthy animal. The transition from the adapted to the maladapted/exhaustion stage is clinically known as the start of the current illness.

Why someone goes from the adapted phase to the maladapted phase is not always obvious. In some people there appears to be no particular reason why asthma should start at a particular age. Maybe the body is just becoming older and less able to keep up successful adaptation. In other cases it appears obvious that 'the straw that broke the camel's back' was an event that produced a temporary excessive stress on the system. In many people, asthma starts soon after a severe attack of flu, glandular fever or a similar virus illness. Childbirth, major operations, and accidents are physically stressful events which can also be the 'final straw'.

Major psychological stresses can also have the same effect. In a study published in the US it was shown that bereavement causes a diminution in the T-lymphocyte count in most people. The level of the T-lymphocytes is possibly one of the better indications of the competence of the immune system to deal with allergic phenomena.

There is a condition called myalgic encephalomyelitis (ME), or chronic fatigue syndrome, which is a severe meningitis-like illness. In a high proportion of cases, after sufferers recover from the primary illness they are never the same again. Many suffer from a wide range of symptoms: fatigue, depression, headaches, nausea and so on. I have treated a lot of these patients and most of their symptoms are related to food allergy or intestinal thrush, and can be eradicated by dealing with these particular problems. I am sure, therefore, that in these people the severe

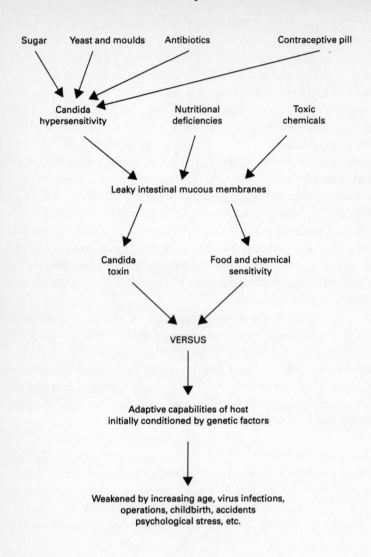

Figure 24 The interrelationship of nutrition, food and chemical and Candida sensitivity to asthma.

vital illness was just a major stressful event which caused them to start to react to dormant food allergies or Candida sensitivity.

Thus, people start to react to foods in the middle part of their lives because of their failure to maintain their adaptation to them. Foods which had appeared to be perfectly innocuous for often 20 to 40 years suddenly become harmful. The whole root of the asthma problem can thus be summarized as shown in Figure 24.

Although everything in Figure 24 is, I believe, basically valid and there is much evidence to support it, there is an awful lot that we still do not know. Most problems can have an explanation at various levels. I have sought to explain allergy in terms of the aggravating or 'insulting' factors and the adaptive reactions of the individual to these. This might be described as the macro-reaction. The micro-reaction – that is, the particulars of the cellular or immunological response – is not at all well understood at the present time. The immunological reaction to most foods is totally unknown. Although a few food reactions are modulated by immunoglobulin E (IgE), the vast majority are not. It is thought that immunoglobulin G, perhaps IgG 4, may be the one that is involved in most food-allergic reactions, but this is pure speculation at the moment.

The fact that we do not yet understand the immunological response, however, does not mean that we cannot adequately deal with it. It could well be 50 years before the details of the immunological response are finally identified. In the mean time there are millions of asthmatic patients who can often be completely cured by the knowledge that is currently available.

Thus, to summarize the basic roots of the allergic response leading to asthma, we have incriminated:

1. Deficiencies of magnesium, vitamins B_{12}, B_6 and vitamin C.
2. A failure of tolerance induction due to exposure to chemicals, many of them inhaled indoors as well as out, combined with a high ingestion of chemicals in foods; these problems occurring at just the same time that we are becoming deficient in the nutrients that are needed to detoxify them.
3. High levels of dust mite induced by effective thermal insulation of houses and consequent high humidity, which encourages the dust mite.
4. The prolific use of sugar, yeast products, the contraceptive pill and antibiotics, predisposing to the Candida hypersensitivity problem.

5. The monotonous, repetitive usage of foods relatively new to the human diet, such as grains, milk, yeasts and sugars.

These traits characterize the living patterns of those Western countries which are showing the great epidemics of asthma. The role of nutrition is, therefore, pivotal in the causation of these conditions, but the straightforward correction of nutritional deficiencies by itself is rarely sufficient to correct the problem. Attention to the subsequent food, chemical and inhalant sensitivities is essential.

16

The Philosophy of the New Approach

The Language and Philosophy of the New Medicine – a New Paradigm?

Unless the reader is familiar with advances in other scientific fields, the work 'paradigm' may not be familiar, but it has entered the English language quite substantially in the past few years. The concept of a paradigm came from *The Structure of Scientific Revolutions* by Thomas H. Kuhn, who described it as a model or a map from which springs a coherent tradition of scientific research. A paradigm has two characteristics: one, it is able to attract an enduring group of adherents away from competing models of scientific activity, and two, it is sufficiently open-ended to leave all sorts of problems to resolve.

The approach that is described in this book is a total revolution in medical thought and is based exclusively on the concept of *cause and effect*. Although many fields of human endeavour, such as engineering, are based solely on isolating causes of problems and dealing fundamentally with those causes, in medicine, except in the area of microbiological disease (bacteria, viruses, fungi, rickettsiae, etc.) this approach has been neglected to an amazing extent.

When I personally meet people unaware of this field, I am usually asked which pill or potion or inhaler I normally use to 'help' asthma. When I reply that I use neither, they usually enquire as to whether I use homoeopathic remedies or Bach flower remedies, and are disappointed to find that I don't use these either. I then attempt to explain that I am trying to seek the cause of the problem and deal with it at source – at which point the bemusement from both lay and professional friends is usually total.

The mental reorientation needed by patients to appreciate the significance of this approach is considerable, but they welcome it since the role of drugs, particularly in relation to asthma, has a poor record. In the case of doctors, the problem is quite enormous as they have had the 'disadvantage' of a medical education – which is one of the most effective brainwashing exercises known to humanity. The reorientation needed by most doctors to understand and appreciate the significance of this subject involves going back to square 1 and starting again in terms of their medical philosophy. This is not easy for conservative people used to diligently travelling in one direction for most of their career. Many physicians find these concepts both challenging and somewhat alarming to their established order of life. Some, therefore, to the consternation of their patients, react with distinct aggression to these concepts.

Most major changes in medical thought and direction have taken about 40–50 years to become generally accepted. In contrast minor changes, such as a new anti-inflammatory drug, are accepted very quickly. The germ theory, for example, was ridiculed by the medical profession in the last century, before it became medical orthodoxy over 30 years after its initial discovery. Other major discoveries, like Harvey's 'circulation of the blood', had similar problems. In 1848, Dr. Ignaz Semmelweis observed that the high death rate from puerperal fever could be reduced dramatically if physicians washed their hands before examining patients and delivering babies. His findings and publications were completely ignored. After a vicious attack on his professional integrity he was ostracized. He died in 1863 after a mental breakdown. His observations and conclusions were correct, of course, but many women and children died needlessly because his colleagues were convinced they had the truth and that his observations had no scientific merit.

The concept of a paradigm, as I stated earlier, came from *The Structure of Scientific Revolutions* by Thomas S. Kuhn. In this treatise, Kuhn describes repeated attacks by the old guard on those who subscribe to new paradigms. When a new paradigm appears in whatever field of science, many (and usually most) of the people in that field cling to the old model or map, but after many years the new map is seen to provide more useful insights and understanding, and the old is gradually discarded. The crisis that leads to a paradigm shift may go on for many decades.

For centuries, many astronomers were unhappy with the Ptolemaic understanding that the earth was fixed, with the moon, sun, planets and stars all revolving around it. Eventually the modern view of Copernicus emerged, that the earth was also a planet revolving around the sun. Over a hundred years elapsed before all astronomers agreed to this new model, and it has remained since then as the accepted paradigm.

Essential to the adoption of a new paradigm is a sense of crisis with the existing model. As yet there is no real sense of crisis within the medical profession, although there is considerable disquiet, particularly in the case of asthma, where the medical profession can only observe a huge and rapidly increasing problem, despite the so-called therapeutic advances that have been made in the past 30 years. If they weren't able to blame it (erroneously) on increasing outdoor pollution there would be a considerable crisis. Amongst patients, however, there is considerable disillusionment with the efforts of the medical profession, as witnessed by the massive growth in alternative and complementary theories such as acupuncture, homoeopathy, reflexology, aromatherapy and traditional Chinese medicine, to mention but a few. The popularity of magazines espousing self-help, and the success of such magazines as *What Doctors Don't Tell You*, which has a splendidly irreverent approach to the medical profession, are also an indication.

There are several reasons why this sense of crisis has not occurred as yet in the medical profession.

- There always seems to be a new wonder drug around the corner.
  There's jam around the corner if not now – the usual slogan of political parties. Rarely does the jam arrive, and if it does it is usually flawed.
- Specialization.
  The increasing trend towards specialization will, I think, in future be seen as one of the most retrograde steps that the medical profession has ever taken. Each specialist examines ever smaller parts of the whole. Patients are passed from specialist to specialist. Specialization is often a classic example of not being able to see the wood for the trees, and the spoof definition of a specialist as someone who knows more and more about less and less, until eventually knowing everything there is to be known about nothing, has a distinct grain of truth in it.
- The psychosomatic explanation gives physicians a blank cheque to absolve themselves from any failure. If the patient doesn't improve with the physician's therapies, it is the patient's fault, and a psychologist is advised. Patients with classic 'respectable' problems, like

asthma, tend to be spared this insult, but it happens all the time with other conditions where there are no obvious visible, radiological or serological (blood) findings.

- Many patients are sensitive to and respectful of their nice, well-intentioned doctors, and are reluctant to criticize them or express their total frustration with their lack of progress.

The existing paradigm in medicine really contains these beliefs about medicine, although its strongest adherents would not categorize them as beliefs, but simply as the way things are.

- The patient *has* asthma. This is in contrast to the idea that this problem has evolved because of certain biochemical, nutritional and environmental factors.
- There is a sharp differentiation between wellness and illness and, if the patient has no radiological or serological findings, he or she is well. There is no sense of a continuum from wellness to illness.
- Adaptation, or the lack of it, is not considered.
- Human bodies are considered sufficiently similar, that for most medical purposes individual differences can be safely ignored.
- Causative factors operate singly, leading to the simplistic statement that exercise is the cause of asthma in certain patients. As exercise does not cause asthma in most people, there must be genetic nutritional and allergic factors at work so that exercise is the final 'straw that breaks the camel's back'.
- Diseases are limited to a single organ and do not imply any dysfunction elsewhere in the body. The patient, for example, has asthma, and that is that.
- There is a limited range of possible causative factors for a disease.
- The mind is capable of causing disease in the body, and is probably the main cause when the disease is poorly understood. Anxiety and tension are known to be able to affect the immune system, but the role of this is probably rather over-played.
- Drugs, despite their known side-effects, may be safely used to treat disease. The idea that the suppression of symptoms in the short term may in the long term be detrimental is ignored (*see Chapter 3*).
- The principles of evolution are not relevant to the practice of medicine.
- Nutrition can be safely ignored, as most people do not suffer from conditions that are caused only by extreme malnutrition.

In contrast, the new paradigm of allergy, environmental and nutritional medicine believes that:

- Symptoms are dynamic because of:
  - (a) variable exposure to food and environmental agents, and
  - (b) variations in immune response.
- There is a continuum ranging from perfect health to death.
- Biochemical individuality is expected. There are huge differences in genetic susceptibility and nutritional status in different patients. There is an optimum nutrition for each individual, and this is frequently much higher than the amount of nutrients required to produce frank nutritional deficiency states.
- Symptoms of disease are caused by breakdowns in complex homeo-static mechanisms, hence causative factors are multiple and very varied. Thus a mythical patient, John Smith, developed the symptoms of asthma in January 1997 as a result of becoming sensitive to several foods and chemicals. This occurred soon after a very acrimonious divorce and worries about the security of his job. The tension and anxiety related to these problems caused a substantial reduction in his T-lymphocytes. His diet at the time was unusually poor as, not wishing to cook, he lived mostly on fast foods with a high chemical and sugar content. As a result there was a demonstrable reduction in his magnesium, zinc and vitamin B status. Because of the fall in these micro-nutrients, his ability to detoxify chemicals was reduced and chemical sensitivity became more manifest.
- Human beings evolve in an environment, and any environmental change which has come in a period of time too short for appropriate evolution to take place must be considered as a possible cause of ill health. Environmental changes require countless generations before the species is able to adapt. Our environment has changed more in the last 100 years than in the rest of history put together, and it will probably take a hundred generations just to adapt to that which has already happened. Thus all drugs, chemicals, electromagnetic radiation and new foods, such as sugar, soy, wheat, etc., are suspect.
- Thus, we believe that:
  - (a) disease does not just happen; the body does not choose to have asthma, headaches, fatigue, joint pains, etc., and
  - (b) the cause of any symptom is theoretically understandable if we know enough about the nutrition, biochemistry and genetic uniqueness of each individual.

This new approach to illness has implications throughout the whole realm of chronic disease. It has been termed environmental medicine, nutritional medicine, allergy, clinical ecology, nutri-allergy, etc., but none of these terms is, by itself, sufficiently wide to embrace the whole field nor to communicate exactly what we do, either with the medical profession, or the public.

In the UK, physicians involved in this area of medicine belong to the British Society for Allergy and Environmental Medicine. In 1993, this Society merged with the British Society for Nutritional Medicine, and both societies, although fully integrated, did for a time retain their original names. The merger was logical and inevitable as it became obvious that chemical sensitivity, for example, was secondary to nutritional factors, and so probably was food sensitivity. Later work showed that even biological inhalant sensitivity could be made worse by magnesium deficiency, affecting the mast cells. In 1996, the two societies agreed on the name the British Society for Allergy, Environmental and Nutritional Medicine.

The Language of Illness

When we think of illness, we usually think of specific disease entities, and these are called diagnoses. A diagnosis ideally tells a lot about an illness. Various acute diseases, such as measles, lend themselves particularly well to this idea. The term 'measles' tells us which micro-organism is causing the problem, the incubation period of the disease, the type of rash that occurs, how long the rash will last, the likely complications, and so on. This same diagnostic philosophy also works well with chickenpox, polio, mumps, whooping cough, etc. Diagnosis is supposed to be aetiological — that is, to explain the cause, and in the examples given above, it does this very satisfactorily.

The specific diagnosis idea, however, works less well with a diagnosis like bronchitis. Bronchitis is an inflammation of the bronchial tubes in the chest, but this inflammation can be caused by a wide range of different germs. Furthermore, the condition occurs only in certain people who are susceptible to the disease, and this susceptibility can be heightened by environmental factors, such as cigarette smoking and industrial pollution. Therefore, one cannot say that any particular germ is the cause of the problem, nor necessarily that it is the cigarette smoking, the industrial pollution, or the individual susceptibility of the host. To say, therefore, that bronchitis causes symptoms of wheezing and coughing is not strictly true.

When we come to most chronic diseases, the 'status and value' of the diagnosis becomes even less significant. This particularly applies to conditions such as asthma. Patients are asked by their physicians to accept the idea that the wheezing in their chest is caused by asthma, which is untrue, as symptoms are not caused by a process named, as in the bronchitis example. Some doctors might reasonably argue that as the cause of asthma is in many cases not known (in their view) such naming performs all the function needed of a diagnostic term. However, talking about the disease as a cause of symptoms leads to treating the disease rather than the patient who is ill. The tendency for doctors to speak and act as if they are treating diseases, not individuals, and the implication that people become ill because they are hapless victims, are two of the most important issues that lie embedded in medical language.

Let us now return to matters discussed earlier. We have seen that individual adverse reaction to foods, chemicals, inhalant particles and the flora of the gut can produce widely varying symptoms in different individuals. Thus, taking a single food, such as milk, we can show it can adversely affect people in many ways, in particular by five well-documented medical statements:

- 'Milk Sensitivity can Produce Asthma', Wraith, D.G., in *Food Allergy & Intolerance* by Brostoff and Challacombe (Bailliere Tindall, 1987).
- 'Milk Sensitivity can Produce Rheumatoid Arthritis', Park, A.C. and Hughes, G.R.V., 'Rheumatoid Arthritis & Food – A Case Study', *British Medical Journal* 282: 2027–29, 1981.
- 'Milk Allergy can Produce Ulcerative Colitis in 20% of Cases with Ulcerative Colitis', Professor Truelove, *British Medical Journal*, 1962.
- 'Milk Allergy can Produce Eczema – A Double Blind Controlled Crossover Trial of Antigen Avoidance Diet in Atopic Eczema', Atherton, D.J. and Soothill, J.F., *Lancet*, 25th February 1978.
- 'Milk Allergy can Produce Migraine – Is Migraine Food Allergy?', Soothill *et al.*, *Lancet*, October 1983.

Thus, adverse reactions to milk can masquerade as a wide variety of symptoms in different people. Similar multiple masquerades can be shown by other foods, chemicals and inhalants, etc. The different guises that reactions to individual items can show is the most practical reason for developing a system of describing signs and symptoms in individuals, which should give us a basis for learning about and treating illness in a way that transcends just naming and treating the symptoms.

The crux of the difference between treating the individual and treating the diagnostic label lies mostly in the consideration given to these symptoms which may seem superfluous to a particular diagnosis.

Symptoms like fatigue, headache, wind, bloating, palpitations, food addiction, excessive sweating, weight gain, adverse responses to alcohol, anal irritation, and improvement on visiting hot, dry climes, are quite extraneous in orthodox medicine to making the diagnosis of asthma. However, as discussed earlier, they are very useful when we are looking at the base causes of allergic wheezing.

Professor Sidney Baker, Research Director of the Gessel Institute of Human Development in Newhaven, Connecticut, has been at the forefront of medical thinking in this area. He has proposed a highly elaborate three-dimensional matrix computer programme which will enable physicians to enter all the sorts of information I have alluded to, to provide an enormous database for progress in this subject. Currently it is being used by all the physicians within the Medical Department of the Gessel Institute.

One way of illustrating the masquerades these various environmental agents can show is to take various classical disease entities and to describe the role that certain basic causes play in them. Some of these 'contributions' have been established in published clinical trials, but many of the associations have been noted by physicians working in the field and used as part of their daily practice. In Figure 25, uninterrupted lines indicate a relationship shown in a published clinical trial; interrupted lines show associations that have been observed but not as yet verified by formal clinical trials.

The lines in the lower part of these diagrams joining the various causes of diseases are entirely based on the clinical experience of physicians and their observations. For instance, the chemical sensitivity usually diminishes or disappears after treatment for Candida. Also, of course, Candida is usually connected with nutritional factors such as high sugar consumption.

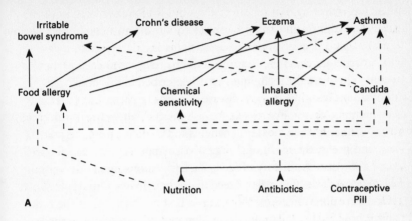

A

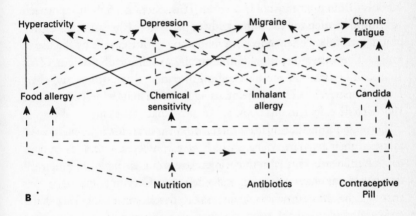

B

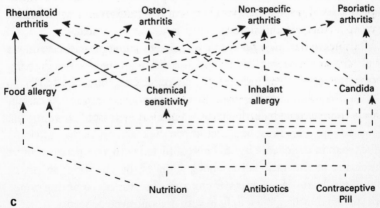

C

Figure 25 Interrelationships of cause and effects

Thus, it is emerging that almost any chronic disease can have almost any cause, and almost any cause can lead to almost any condition. The logical way of dealing with these problems is, therefore, to diagnose which particular causative factor(s) could be relevant in each particular patient. These are the techniques I have described in this book.

Physicians who like to view disease in terms of cause and effect have been naturally drawn, like myself, to this subject. Many other doctors are, however, uneasy when looking at patients and medicine from this point of view, and prefer the traditional organ-based approach. In fact, for well over 2,000 years the history of medicine has demonstrated this constant schism between the two major directions of thought and philosophy.

One direction of medical thought can best be described as the rationalist school, and at the moment this dominates the teaching at medical schools throughout most of the world. This school prefers the approach of knowledge derived from the study of pathology (the study of organs, blood, etc.) followed by symptom suppression, for example by the use of drugs. The other direction is the empirical school of thought. This approach is based on the observation of patients' symptoms and their interaction with the environment, using the term in its widest sense. The approach described in this book is, of course, that of the empirical school.

Throughout medical history these two main currents of thought have followed their separate courses, which have conflicted with and yet have exerted influence on each other. There are some examples of empirical thought in rationalist teaching and vice versa. Certainly, the rationalist approach has brought about many major advances in medicine, but the biggest advance of all, the germ concept of disease, was initially an empirical idea which was strongly resisted for many years by the medical establishment of the day. Bacteria and viruses are, of course, external environmental agents, and their effect on human beings is now well accepted.

Sir Francis Bacon, who was a founder of modern science and an empiricist, believed that the purpose of science was to observe, describe and characterize the processes of nature, rather than necessarily to explain them. Hippocrates made the empirical observation that certain people were harmed by eating cheese, but most were not. Therefore, he reasoned that there must be something in the reactivity of the individual rather than in the cheese itself. This conflicted with a tendency of most physicians of the rationalist school, initiated by Aristotle, to prefer pathological knowledge over symptomatic observations, ignoring symptoms unless they happened to fit in with preconceived concepts.

My rationalist medical school education taught me to focus my attention on specific disease entities and on pathological findings, especially objective laboratory findings. It was necessary to find something wrong with the patient with objective tests in order to have a 'rational basis for treatment'. The treatment then took the direction of opposing, combating or suppressing symptoms with analgesic drugs, anti-spasmodic drugs, anti-inflammatory drugs, anti-bronchospasm drugs, corticosteroids and so on.

In the last century Constantine Hering taught that the suppression of acute illness tends to promote chronic illness. He also taught that the natural processes of healing functioned best when the physician promoted the reversion of chronic symptoms to acute symptoms. In this respect Hering foresaw the basic concept of our approach: that a return to health requires an initial clearing of the chronic adaptive state (as, for example, on the 5–6 day hypoallergenic diet), after which time chronic symptoms can revert to acute symptoms (Rinkel's hyperacute response). At this stage the various excitants can be identified.

Most physicians, because of the training which directs their attention, beliefs and behaviour to the rationalist approach, find it difficult to accept empirical approaches and regard them as unscientific or not being within the scope of the practice of medicine. An example of this is the role of cigarette smoking in the causation of lung cancer, a classic instance of an environmental stimulus causing a disease process. In 1958 I was a medical student and, having reviewed all the clinical papers supporting this view, I discussed the matter with several consultants at my medical school. In view of the weight of evidence, I wanted to know why the fact that cigarette smoking was a cause of lung cancer was not at that time being taught at my medical school. I was told that, if I believed that cigarette smoking was a cause of lung cancer, I was mad. That lung cancer could be caused by an environmental agent such as a simple cigarette was beyond belief. These physicians were much more interested in teaching the various histological forms that cancer could take, rather than the environmental agents that could cause it.

In fact, there is an inherent desire on the part of most scientists to prefer complex research to simple research. They would argue that only by complex research into the intricate details of bodily functions can we gain an overall picture of disease processes, and only then can we succeed in combating disease. Such an argument has inherent flaws. In most cases, bodily mechanisms are so complex that it will take many decades or many centuries to understand them properly. The problem resembles an underground system of such vastness that, as soon as one channel is charted, two or three new ones are discovered. This rationalist-inspired complex research is, therefore, likely to be a very long-term saga with no guarantee of anything useful emanating at the end of it. Simple research into the interrelationship of lung cancer and cigarette smoking has yielded enormous practical benefits in indicating the value of stopping this habit. Many thousands of lives have already been saved as a result of this research.

In contrast to the above, complex research such as gene regulation of the metabolism of the thousands of chemicals in tobacco smoke and their effect on the human body has been of minute value.

One of the interesting things about medicine is that it is often hard to establish the specific time that a new concept has become generally acceptable. In which year, for example, was it finally accepted that cigarette smoking was the main cause of lung cancer? Possibly about 12 years ago, as I do not remember any concerted arguments to the contrary being advanced in the last 10 years. There is, in truth, no particular point in time. As Dr. Ronald Finn once told me, there are four stages in the development of a new medical idea:

Stage 1: You are mad.
Stage 2: I suppose there might be something in it.
Stage 3: There could be something in it, but where is the proof?
Stage 4: Well, of course, we knew all along.

Thus, this approach represents a new paradigm with a new language expressing medical thought, and an emphasis on empirical observation and thought instead of the rationalist school of thought. The adoption of these ideas is liable to be slow and strongly resisted because of the innate conservatism and herd instincts of the medical profession, and the vested interests of the pharmaceutical industry, some sections of which have shown a tendency to attack any form of non-drug medicine. There is an extensive account of this is the book entitled *Dirty Medicine* by Martin Shaw (Slingshot Publications). For all these reasons it is likely that most physicians will cling to the existing paradigm for a long time. But even when there is a transfer to the new paradigm, no model will give the answers to all problems. Doubtless, in decades to come the new paradigm may be supplanted by another model or map which will reveal further insights into how human beings can rid themselves of the disease processes that ruin so many of our lives.

Summary

This book describes the allergy, environmental and nutritional approach to solving the problem of asthma. It is an approach based solely on sorting out cause and effect, and describes methods for dealing with the causes of asthma at their source. This approach is not aimed at relieving asthma, or helping asthma, or modifying its worse effects. It is aimed at *solving the problem*.

Apart from the use of some nutritional supplements, and possibly anti-fungal drugs in a small proportion of cases, the approach does not involve using pills, potions, inhalers, nebulizers, steroids or amino-phylline injections, or any other symptom-suppressant drug. Nor does it rely on homoeopathic remedies, aromatherapy, Chinese medicine, herbal medicine, naturopathy, reflexology, shiatsu, or any other alternative medical strategy. The ideas in this book are not as yet taught at medical schools, apart from information that reactions to dust, dust mite, moulds, pollens and animal danders are major causes of asthma. Nevertheless, most of the evidence relating to this subject has been published in individual articles in main line medical journals, as witness all the references scattered throughout this book. Most of the main players in this medical saga, both in the UK, US, Canada and Australia, are hospital-based consultants or ex-general practitioners. In the US a high proportion of the practitioners are Board-Certified Allergists or Board-Certified ENT Specialists.

Thus, although these strategies, as a cohesive whole, are not well understood through mainstream medicine, its practitioners consider themselves more closely allied to traditional medicine than to alternative medicine. In truth, the subject at the moment is in a sort of no-man's land; not main line medicine and not alternative medicine.

In general we have not sought to publish work relating to this subject in books devoted to alternative medical strategies such as homoeopathy, aromatherapy, naturopathy, Chinese medicine, etc., as this would make it difficult for the subject to be assimilated into main line medicine, where we hope it will become the medicine of the 21st century.

I elected to write this book on asthma, but in truth similar books could be written describing the same approach in relation to eczema, urticaria, irritable bowel, Crohn's disease, rhinitis, chronic fatigue states, endogenous depression, hyperactivity in children, and several other chronic medical disorders.

In 1986 I wrote a similar book entitled *The Migraine Revolution* which described this approach as it relates to migraine. In 1990 came *Arthritis – The Allergy Connection*, which described the use of this approach in all forms of arthritis, but especially rheumatoid arthritis. In 1995 I considerably updated this latter book and added a lot of nutritional information, and the title was changed to *Arthritis – Allergy, Nutrition and the Environment*. All three of these books are published by Thorsons.

However, in asthma we probably have the clearest evidence of the interplay of nutritional factors, biological inhalant sensitivities, chemical sensitivities, Candida hypersensitivity and food intolerance going on to produce the symptoms which are called asthma.

Another way of describing these problems is to write a book, for example, on food sensitivity or chemical sensitivity and to examine its role in many diseases. This is rather like looking through one or the other end of the same telescope. In fact, most of the books currently available are written from this general viewpoint and not from the specific viewpoint of the disease process. Many of these books are excellent and have done a great deal to increase general awareness of this subject. The problem with these books is that many patients suffering with specific diseases such as eczema, irritable bowel, Crohn's disease, migraine, etc. may not really realize that their own problems have anything to do with, for example, food sensitivity. Even if they do, food sensitivity represents only a part of the problem and not the whole problem.

Every week I see an article in the lay or professional press where some so-called expert states that asthma is clearly to do with the Western way of life and that it is increasing all the time. Poorly informed sources, like some politicians, are happy to put the whole blame on outdoor air pollution and suggest draconian measures against the motor car. However, as there is more asthma in children on the Isle of Skye where there is virtually no outdoor air pollution than in Aberdeen or Cardiff where there is a lot, the eradication of motor vehicle exhaust fumes is hardly likely to solve the problem. The highest echelons of the medical profession are agreed that outdoor air pollution plays only a small role in this sorry saga, but it has not been generally appreciated as yet that indoor air pollution through a lethal cocktail of chemicals and dustmites is the major cause of this condition. The amount of nitrogen dioxide produced in the average kitchen far exceeds the pollution on even the busiest city street. Large amounts of formaldehyde and other chemicals, and 'outgas' from woollen carpets laid wall-to-wall in many houses, are aggravated by the effective thermal insulation of most homes.

Serious consideration should be given to reducing the indoor chemical pollution of our homes and electric ovens should be preferred to gas. Gas and oil boilers should preferably be installed outside the house. In homes where this is impossible, electric storage heaters would appear to be the best answer.

Floor coverings which do not emit chemicals, such as terrazo tiles, marble, hard woods, etc. are ideal, but synthetic carpets are less of a problem than wool. The rubber underlay can also be a problem for some asthma sufferers.

Measures to reduce dust mite exposure in thermally insulated homes, in which the humidity is not allowed to escape, include dehumidifiers, effective vacuum cleaners, mattress and pillow enclosures, acaracide sprays for carpets and liquid nitrogen treatment for mattresses, pillows and carpets.

Nutritionally, one's status of magnesium and certain B-vitamins should be determined. If magnesium status is deficient it should be corrected. The junk food diet eaten unquestioningly by so much of our population should be abandoned. The monotonous repetitive diet of bread and other cereals, sugar, soy, yeast and milk, almost inevitably leads to food sensitivity in many people. These are all 'new' foods in our diet and we have had a relatively short period of time to get used to them. As a species we have, for over a hundred thousand years, eaten vegetables, fruits, berries, nuts, meats and fish, and many of the population, especially children, eat very little of these foods to which we have become well adapted.

As emphasized throughout this book, the particular cause of each individual's asthma varies a lot and it is essential to sort out the causes on an individual basis.

Perhaps the most disappointing thing in the past few years is the stubborn resistance of the medical profession (with a few very notable exceptions) to look seriously at the enormous potential of intradermal neutralization treatment to desensitize people to inhaled allergens such as dust, dust mites, moulds and pollens. Certainly the old-fashioned incremental desensitization was pretty unpopular, and for very good reasons, the best one of which was that it worked for only about one person in six. Most physicians stopped using it because there was a handful of deaths in severe asthmatics. Incremental desensitization has given the whole concept of desensitization a bad name, and most physicians haven't any idea of the differences that are offered by neutralization treatment.

In Chapters 12 and 13 I have explained that the neutralizing doses employed are individual to each patient. The doses are those which give a negative skin response and immediately tend to make the patient feel improved, in contrast to incremental desensitization where each injection was often followed by an asthmatic attack. In practice, the doses used are several hundred times weaker than those employed in incremental desensitization, and despite several decades of use by several thousand physicians worldwide there has not been as yet a single fatality recorded. There is *no* drug that can match this safety record. The technique has been evaluated in a large number of clinical trials, mentioned in Chapter 14.

One of the most unfortunate side-effects of the abandonment by many physicians of any form of desensitization is that most now do not even do the elementary prick tests which have been used for many years. The argument is that if desensitization is not to be employed, there is not much point in establishing which allergies are involved as the treatment is going to be symptom-suppressive drugs, which will work to some extent whatever the basic cause of the problem. In Chapter 3 I have discussed the role of these drugs in perpetuating and generally making the problems worse in the long term. In that chapter I quoted specific trials showing that beta-2 agonist inhalers, such as Ventolin, are a good idea in the short term but make the condition worse in the long run. The whole history of drug suppression of asthma over the last 50 years has been a catalogue of one disaster after another, with many dead patients along the way.

If someone is driving a car and notices the oil-warning light has come on, there are two possible courses of action: replenish the oil in the engine or put a sticking plaster over the light so that the driver will no longer see and worry about the lack of oil. Symptoms can be fairly looked at as a warning light of underlying biochemical disorder. Drug suppression of these symptoms leads to disregard of the underlying causes and, as in the case of the oil-deficient car, the problem is likely to get worse. As Constantine Hering taught in the 19th century, the suppression of acute illness leads to chronic illness.

Determining cause and effect in human illness is enormously cost-effective, as opposed to the standard techniques involving constant ingestion of drugs, and frequent hospitalization. Governments world-wide have become increasingly worried by the escalating cost of medicine. The problem is probably at its worst in the US, where medical services in 1992 cost the American people $817 billion.[1] According to the President of the Institute for Healthcare Improvement in Boston, if this vast sum of money, 14 per cent of the US Gross National Product, was distributed to all the children born in the USA in 1992, it would buy each of them a full college education, two medium-sized homes and a Rolls Royce. This sum is also, incidentally, about £100 billion in excess of the Gross National Product of Italy. Americans are terrified by the potential cost of their future medical care, and many have already been crippled financially. The trend continues to increase annually.

In the UK, medicine is grabbing an ever-increasing part of the Gross National Product. In 1994 it was round about 8 per cent, and the NHS is costing about 3 per cent more each year in real terms than in the preceding year. Any government of any political hue will have to take measures to limit this growth, which national economies cannot ultimately sustain. Many asthmatics cost the state more than £50,000 spread over many years. Most patients using the techniques described in this book would cost themselves or the state much less than £1,000. Having ever more doctors prescribing ever more drugs with ever more side-effects, ever more hospitalization and ever-escalating costs, is a prescription for disaster.

Several thousand patients in the UK alone, and some hundreds of thousands of patients in the US, have already had their asthma problems reversed. Sometimes this has occurred in as short a period as a few days or a few weeks. Many physicians have been impressed by these recoveries and are sending their patients to have this form of treatment. However, interesting one physician after another is a painfully slow way of disseminating this type of knowledge. What is required is further evaluation of this approach by the highest echelons of the medical establishment.

The asthma epidemic is a man-made phenomenon and if man can make it he can surely 'un-make' it. Countless people, and especially children, are suffering unnecessarily from this epidemic. It is surely now time that we adopt the sort of measures outlined in this book to reverse this major aberration that has occurred in the second half of the 20th century.

Useful Addresses

Medical Organizations

Airedale Allergy Centre
High Hall
Steeton
Airedale
Keighley
W Yorks BD20 6SB
01535 656013

Allergolab Research
(Dr. K. Eaton)
Templars
Terrace Road South
Binfield
Berks RG12 5DN
01344 53919
01344 306280 (fax)

Biolab Medical Unit
The Stonehouse
9 Weymouth Street
London W1N 3FF
0171 636 5959
0171 580 3910 (fax)

Dr. S. Birtwistle
66 Station Road
Fulbourn
Cambs CB1 5ES
01223 880777

Breakspear Hospital
Belswains Lane
Hemel Hempstead
Herts HP3 9HP
01442 61333
01442 66388 (fax)

The Burghwood Clinic
(Dr. J. Mansfield)
34 Brighton Road
Banstead
Surrey SM7 1BS
01737 361177
01737 352245 (fax)

Department of Immunology
(Dr. J. Brostoff)
Middlesex Hospital
Mortimer Street
London W1N 8AA
0171 380 9351

Forestside Medical Practice
(Dr. M. Radcliffe)
Old Malthouse
Main Road
Marchwood
Southampton SO40 4UZ
01703 871233

Dr. Stewart Morison
72 Francis Avenue
Southsea
Portsmouth PO4 0HP
01705 296145

Salford Private Allergy Centre
(Dr. D. Freed)
14 Marston Road
Salford
Manchester M7 4ER
0161 795 6225

Sozo Clinic
(Dr. H. Cox)
14 Ayleswater
Watermead
Buckingham Road
Aylesbury
Bucks HP11 3FB
01296 399317

Dr. D. West & Dr. E. Hamlyn
Ivybridge Allergy Testing Centre
Rutt House
Ivybridge
Devon PL21 0DQ
01752 892792

Support Groups

Local allergy support groups are usually listed in the reference sections of local public libraries.

UK

Action Against Allergy
P.O. Box 278
Twickenham
Middx TW1 4QQ
0181 744 1171

British Society for Allergy, Environmental & Nutritional Medicine (BSAENM)
Secretary

Acorns
Romsey Road
Cadnam
Southampton SO4 2NN
01703 812124
01703 813 912 (fax)

Food & Chemical Allergy Association
27 Ferringham Lane
Ferring-by-Sea
West Sussex BN12 5NB
01903 241178

**Hythe Food & Chemical
Victims' Allergy Club**
44 Fairview Drive
Hythe
Southampton
(No telephone enquiries)

**National Society for Research
into Allergy**
P.O. Box 45
Hinckley
Leics LE10 1JY
01455 851546

**Oxford Group for Management
of Food Intolerance**
01865 552824

US

**American Academy of
Environmental Medicine**
4510 West 89th Street
Suite 110
Prairie Village
Kansas 66207–2282
913 642 6062
913 341 6912 (fax)

**The Human Ecology Research
Foundation**
505 North Lake Shore Drive
Suite 6506
Chicago, Illinois 60611

**Alan Mandell Center for
Bio-Ecologic Diseases**
3 Brush Street
Norwalk, Connecticut 06850

Australia

Allergy Association of Australia
P.O. Box 298
Ringwood
Victoria 3134
03 720 3215

**Allergy and Intolerant
Reactions Association**
P.O. Box 1780
Canberra City 2601

**Allergy Recognition &
Management**
P.O. Box 2
Sandy Bay
Tasmania 7005
002 236 797

New Zealand

Allergy Awareness Association
P.O. Box 120701
Penrose
Auckland 6

Republic of Ireland

Irish Allergy Association
P.O. Box 1967
Churchtown
Dublin 14

Useful Suppliers

UK

Allerayde
3 Sanigar Court
Whittle Close
Newark
Notts NG24 2BW
01636 613444
01636 611186 (fax)

Allergy Relief Products Ltd
Mansion House
14 Mansion Road
Southampton SO15 3BP
01703 224793
01703 332919 (fax)

Arco Limited
P.O. Box 21
Waverley Street
Hull
Humberside HU1 2SJ
01482 27678
01482 218536 (fax)

Beta Plus Limited
177 Haydons Road
London SW19 8TB
0181 543 1142
0181 543 4317 (fax)

C.B.C.
215 Carshalton Road
Carshalton
Surrey SM5 3PZ
0181 770 7646
Suppliers of liquid nitrogen

Crawford Pharmaceuticals
Furtho House,
20 Towcester Road
Old Stratford,
Milton Keynes
Herts MK19 6AQ
01908 262346
01928 567730 (fax)

Foodwatch International Limited
9 Corporation Street
Taunton
Somerset TA1 4AJ
01823 325022

General Dietary Limited
P.O. Box 38
Kingston Upon Thames
Surrey KT2 7YP
0181 336 2323
0181 942 8274 (fax)

Healthy Buildings International Ltd
Wyvols Court
Swallowfield
Berks RG7 1PY
01734 880248
01734 880360 (fax)

The Healthy House
Cold Harbour
Ruscombe, Stroud
Glos GL6 6DA
01453 752216
01453 753533 (fax)

Honeywell Envirocare Air Filters
0800 345000

Larkhall Green Farm
225 Putney Bridge Road
London SW15 2PY
0181 874 1130
0181 871 0066 (fax)

The Linen Cupboard
21–22 Great Castle Street
London W1N 7AA
0171 629 4062

Medivac plc
Bollin House
Riverside Works
Manchester Road
Wilmslow
Cheshire SK9 1BE
01625 539401
01625 539507 (fax)

Mountain Breeze Ltd
6 Priorswood Place
Skelmersdale
Lancs WN8 9QB
01695 21155

Nilfisk Limited
Newmarket Road
Bury St Edmunds
Suffolk IP33 3SR
0800 252 296

The Real Meat Company Limited
East Hill Farm
Heytesbury
Warminster
Wilts BA12 0HR
01985 840436
01985 840243

C. D. Searle & Co. Ltd
Freepost
P.O. Box 53
Lane End Road
High Wycombe
Bucks HP12 3BR
01494 21124

Slumberland plc
Salmon Fields
Royton
Oldham
Lancs OL2 6SB
0161 628 2898

Australia

Allergy Aid Centre
1st Floor
Pran Central
325 Chapel Street
Prahran
Victoria 3181
03 529 7348

Country Harvest Products
*Address as opposite – National
Dietary Supplies*

National Dietary Supplies
2A/23 Koornang Road
Carnegie
Victoria 3163
03 563 6538

References

Chapter 1

1. V. Serafini, 'Can fatal asthma be prevented? – a personal view', *Clinical Exp Allergy* 22 (1992): 576–88.
2. W. Osler, *The Principles and Practice of Medicine* (Edinburgh: Young J. Pentland, 1892): 500.
3. H. A. Christian and J. Mackenzie (eds), *The Oxford Textbook of Medicine* (Oxford University Press, 1920): 232.
4. F. Coke, *Asthma* (Bristol: Wright & Sons, 1923): 104.
5. J. J. Conybeare, *A Textbook of Medicine* (Edinburgh: Livingstone, 1929): 486.
6. P. G. J. Burney, 'Strategy for asthma', *British Medical Journal* 303 (1991): 571–3; M. R. Sears, 'Epidemiology of asthma', in D. C. Flenley and T. L. Petty (eds), *Recent Advances in Respiratory Medicine* (vol 4; Edinburgh: Churchill Livingstone, 1986): 1–11; T. Haahtela, H. Lindholm, F. Bjorksten, K. Koskenvuo and L. Laitinen, 'Prevalence of asthma in Finnish young men', *British Medical Journal* 301 (1990): 266–8; P. G. J. Burney, S. Chinn and R. J. Rona, 'Has the prevalence of asthma increased in children? Evidence from the national survey of health and growth', *British Medical Journal* 300 (1990): 1306–10; A. L. Sheffer, quoted by B. Zweiman in open letter to members of the American Academy of Allergy and Immunology, July 1991; J. Crane, N. Pearce, R. Beasley and C. Burgess, 'Worldwide worsening of wheezing – is the cure the cause?' *Lancet* 339 (1992): 814; A. Khot and R. Burn, 'Deaths from asthma', *British Medical Journal* 289 (1984): 557; R. M. Sly, 'Increases in deaths from asthma', *Ann Allergy* 53 (1984): 20–5; D. I. Mullaly, W. A. Howard, T. J. Hubbard, J. S. Grauman and S. G. Cohen, 'Increased hospitalisations for asthma among children in

the Washington DC area during 1961–1981', *Ann Allergy* 53 (1984): 15–19; R. A. Shaw, J. Crane and T. V. O'Donnell, 'Prevalence of asthma in children', *British Medical Journal* 300 (1990): 1652–3; C. F. Robertson, E. Heycock, J. Bishop, T. Nolan, A. Olinsky and P. D. Phelan, 'Prevalence of asthma in Melbourne in school children: changes over 26 years', *British Medical Journal* 302 (1991): 1116–18.

7. A. L. Sheffer, 'International Consensus on Diagnosis and Treatment of Asthma', *Clinical Exp Allergy* 22 suppl. 1 (1992): xi.

8. Jane Austin, 'Prevalence of asthma and wheeze in the Highlands of Scotland', *Archives of Diseases in Childhood* 71 (1994): 211–16.

9. 'Prevalence of asthma and allergy disorders among children in United Germany. A descriptive comparison', *British Medical Journal* 305 (1992): 305–1395.

10. T. Randolph, *Human Ecology and Susceptibility to the Chemical Environment* (Springfield, IL: Charles C. Thomas, 1962).

11. Sheffer, 'International Consensus', *op cit.*

12. F. Godlee and A. Walker, 'Importance of a Health Environment', *British Medical Journal* 303 (1991): 1124–6.

13. R. Robinson, 'Wheezy children', *British Medical Journal* 302 (1991): 1516.

14. J. Rees, 'Beta-2 antagonists and asthma' (editorial), *British Medical Journal* 302 (1991): 1166–7.

15. Crane, Pearce, Beasley and Burgess, *op cit.*

16. N. Pearce, 'End of the New Zealand asthma mortality epidemic', *Lancet* 345 (1995): 41.

17. J. Crane *et al.*, 'Prescribed fenoterol and death from asthma in New Zealand 1981–1983. A case control study', *Lancet* 1 (1989): 917–22.

18. E. H. Brunner *et al.*, 'Effect of parentral magnesium on pulmonary function, plasma C-amp, and histamine in bronchial asthma', *Journal Asthma* 22 (1985): 3; H. Okayama *et al.*, 'Bronchodilating effect of intravenous magnesium sulphate in bronchial asthma', *Journal of the American Medical Association* 257 (1987): 1076; E. M. Skobeloff *et al.*, 'Intravenous magnesium sulphate for the treatment of acute asthma in the emergency department', *Journal of the American Medical Association* 282 (1989): 1210.

19. 'A synergism of antigen challenge and severe magnesium deficiency on blood and urinary histamine levels in rats', *Journal of the American College of Nutrition* 9.6 (1990): 616–22.

20. D. Wraith, in Brostoff and Challacombe (eds), *Food Allergy and Intolerance* (Philadelphia: Ballière Tindall, 1987).
21. C. Infant-Rivarde, 'Childhood asthma and indoor environmental factors', *American Journal of Epidemiology* 137 (1993): 834–44.

Chapter 2

1. P. G. J. Burney, S. Chinn and R. J. Rona, 'Has the prevalence of asthma increased in children? Evidence from the national survey of health and growth', *British Medical Journal* 300 (1990): 1306–10.
2. H. Anderson, 'Increase in hospital admissions for childhood asthma; trends in referral, severity and readmissions from 1970 to 1989 in a health region of the UK', *Thorax* 44 (1989): 614–19.
3. A. L. Burr, 'Changes in asthma prevalence: two surveys 15 years apart', *Archives of Diseases in Childhood* 64 (1989): 1452–56.
4. D. M. Fleming, 'Prevalence of asthma and hay fever in England and Wales', *British Medical Journal* 294 (1987): 279.
5. Peat *et al.*, 'Changing prevalence of asthma in Australian children, *British Medical Journal* 308 (1994): 1591–6.
6. C. F. Robertson, E. Heycock, J. Bishop, T. Nolan, A. Olinsky and P. D. Phelan, 'Prevalence of asthma in Melbourne in school children: changes over 26 years', *British Medical Journal* 302 (1991): 1116–18.
7. M. Flynn, 'Respiratory symptoms; bronchial reactivity and atopy in Fijian and Indian children, *American Journal Respiratory Crit Care Med* (in press).
8. C. Robertson, 'International comparison of asthma prevalence in children, Australia, Switzerland, Chile', *Paediatric Pulmonal* 16 (1993): 219–26.
9. N. Pearce, 'End of the New Zealand asthma mortality epidemic', *Lancet* 345 (1995): 41.
10. T. Haahtela, H. Lindholm, F. Bjorksten, K. Koskenvuo and L. Laitinen, 'Prevalence of asthma in Finnish young men', *British Medical Journal* 301 (1990): 266–8.

Chapter 3

1. N. Pearce, 'End of the New Zealand asthma mortality epidemic', *Lancet* 345 (1995): 41.
2. R. L. Benson and Pearlman, 'Clinical effects of epinephrine by inhalation', *J Allergy* 19 (1948): 129–40.
3. J. Crane *et al.*, 'Prescribed fenoterol and death from asthma in New Zealand 1981–1983. A case control study', *Lancet* (1989): 917–22.
4. Pearce, *op cit.*
5. B. Pipworth, 'Bronchodilator subsensitivity to salbutamol after twice daily salmeterol in asthmatic patients', *Lancet* 346 (1995): 201–6.
6. Cockcroft, 'Regular inhaled salbutamol and airway responsiveness to allergen', *Lancet* 342 (1993): 833.
7. *New England Journal of Medicine*, Feb. 20th, 1992.
8. *Journal of Allergy and Clinical Immunology* 76 (1985).
9. S. Capewell, 'Purpura and dermal thinning associated with high-dose inhaled corticosteroids', *British Medical Journal* 300 (1990): 1548.
10. *Lancet* 6 (July 1991).
11. K. Horsefield, 1981, cited by C. T. Buckey, 'The Role of Bronchial Musculature', *Lancet* ii (1989): 836–37.

Chapter 6

1. D. G. Wraith, 'Asthma and rhinitis', *Clinical Immunology Allergy* 2 (1982): 101–12.
2. A. H. Rowe, 'Bronchial asthma because of food and inhalant allergy and less frequent drug and chemical allergy', in *idem, Food Allergy* (Springfield, IL: Charles C. Thomas, 1972): 169–210.
3. J. W. Gerrard, 'Food induced respiratory disease', in J. W. Gerrard (ed.), *Food Allergy: New Perspectives* (Springfield, IL: Charles C. Thomas, 1980): 85–98.
4. K. A. Oggle and J. D. Bullock, 'Children with allergic rhinitis and bronchial asthma treated with elimination diet. A five-year follow up', *Ann Allergy* 44 (1980): 273–8.

5. N. Papageorgiou *et al.*, 'Neutrophil activity, chemotactic activity in milk induced asthma', *Journal Allergy and Clin Immunology* 72 (1983): 75–82.
6. W. T. Kniker *et al.*, 'Non IgE mediated and delayed adverse reactions to food or additives', in J. B. Brenoman (ed.), *Handbook on Food Allergies* (New York: Muriel Decker, 1985).
7. R. Dahl, Zeteerstrom, 'The effect of orally administered sodium chromoglycate on allergic reactions caused by food allergens', *Clin Allergy* 8 (1978): 419–22.
8. R. Dahl, 'Oral and inhaled sodium chromoglycate in challenge tests with food allergens or acetysalicylic acid', *Allergy* 36 (1981): 161–5.
9. B. Stenius and Lemola, 'Hypersensitivity to acetyl salicylic acid and tartrazine in patients with asthma', *Clin Allergy* 6 (1976): 119–29.
10. B. J. Freedman, 'Asthma induced by sulphur dioxide, benzoate and tartrazine contained in orange drinks', *Clin Allergy* 7 (1977): 407–15.
11. B. J. Freedman, 'Sulphur dioxide in foods and beverages. Its use in preservatives and its effects on asthma', *British Journal Dis Chest* 14 (1980): 128–34.
12. G. T. Baker *et al.*, 'Bronchospasm induced by metabisulphite containing food, and drugs', *Med Journal Aust* ii (1981): 614–16.
13. Stevenson and Simon, 'Sensitivity to ingested metabisulphites in asthmatic subjects', *J Allergy and Clin Immunology* 68 (1981): 26–32.
14. Ortolani *et al.*, 'Diagnosis of intolerances to food additives', *Ann Allergy* 53 (1984): 587–91.

Chapter 7

1. C. Infant-Rivarde, 'Childhood asthma and indoor environmental factors, *American Journal of Epidemiology* 137 (1993): 834–44.
2. Tunnicliffe, 'Effect of domestic concentrations of nitrogen dioxide on airway responses to inhaled allergens in asthmatic patients', *Lancet* 344 (1994): 1733–36.
3. A. L. Devalia, 'Effect of nitrogen dioxide and sulphur dioxide on airway response of mild asthmatic patients to allergen inhalation', *Lancet* 344 (1994): 1668–71.

4. Jarvis, 'Association of respiratory symptoms and lung function in young adults with use of domestic gas appliances', *Lancet* 347 (1996): 426.

5. D. P. Harlos, 'Acute exposure to nitrogen dioxide during cooking or commuting'. Dissertation, Harvard School of Public Health, Boston, MA, 1988.

6. J. M. Samet *et al.*, 'Nitrogen dioxide and respiratory illness in infants, *American Review Respir Disease* 148 (1933): 1258–65.

7. G. F. T. Brought, 'Air Quality in the UK. A summary of results from instrumented air monitoring networks in 1991–1992', Warren Spring Laboratory report LR 941 (Stevenage WSL, 1993).

8. Dr C. Shim, *American Journal of Medicine* 80 (1980).

9. Norbäck, 'Asthmatic symptoms and volatile organic compounds, formaldehyde and carbon dioxide in dwellings', *Occupational and Environmental Medicine* 52 (1995): 388–95.

10. R. Stankus *et al.*, 'Cigarette smoke sensitive asthma challenge studies', *Journal of Allergy and Clinical Immunology* 82 (3 part 1; 1988): 331–8.

11. D. Strachan, 'Incidence and prognosis of asthma and wheezing illness from early childhood to age 33 in a National British Cohort', *British Medical Journal* 312 (1996): 1195–99.

12. Jane Austin, 'Prevalence of asthma and wheeze in the Highlands of Scotland', *Archives of Diseases in Childhood* 71 (1994): 211–16.

13. J. R. Greer, 'Asthma related to occupational and ambient air pollution in non-smokers', *J Occup Environmental Medicine* 35 (1993): 909–15.

14. W. J. S. T. Matthias, 'Road traffic and adverse effects on respiratory health in children', *British Medical Journal* 307 (1993): 596–600.

15. Austin, *op cit.*

16. 'Prevalence of asthma and atopy in two areas of West and East Germany', *American J Respir Crit Care Med* 149 (1994): 358–64.

17. B. J. Freedman, 'Asthma induced by sulphur dioxide, benzoate and tartrazine contained in orange drinks', *Clin Allergy* 7 (1977): 407–15.

18. *Ibid.*; R. Bush *et al.*, 'A critical evaluation of clinical trials in reactions to sulphites', *Journal of Allergy and Clinical Immunology* 78 (1986): 191–202; D. Wraith, 'Asthma', in Brostoff and Challacombe (eds), *Food Allergy and Intolerance* (Philadelphia: Ballière Tindall, 1987): 486–97.

19. D. Allen *et al.*, 'Monosodium L glutamate induced asthma', *Journal of Allergy and Clinical Immunology* 80 (4; 1987): 530–7.

Chapter 8

1. J. Savolainen, 'Candida albicans and chronic dermatitis', *Clinical and Experimental Allergy* 23 (1993): 332–9; G. Holti, 'Candida allergy', Wm Winner HI ED, Symposium on Candida Infections (Edinburgh & London: E & S Livingstone, 1966): 74–81; James J. Warin, 'An assessment of the role of Candida albicans and food yeasts in chronic urticaria', *British Journal of Dermatology* 84 (1971): 227–37; Rosenberg *et al.*, 'Oral nystatin in the treatment of psoriasis', *Arch of Dermatology* 120 (1984): 433.

2. D. Atherton, 'A double-blind controlled cross-over trial of an antigen avoidance diet in atopic eczema', *Lancet* (25th Feb 1978): 401.

3. 'Double-blind controlled trial of effect of house dust mite allergen avoidance on atopic dermatitis', *Lancet* 347 (1996): 15–18.

4. Savolainen, *op cit.*

5. Orion Truss, 'Tissue injury induced by Candida albicans. Mental and neurological manifestations', *Journal of orthomolecular Psychiatry* 7.1; 'Restoration of immunologic competence to Candida albicans', *Journal of Orthomolecular Psychiatry* 9.4; 'The role of Candida albicans in human illness', *Journal of Orthomolecular Psychiatry* 10.4.

6. I. H. Itkin and M. Dennis, 'Bronchial hypersensitivity to extracts of Candida albicans', *Journal of Allergy* 37 (1966): 187–95.

7. P. Gumowski, 'Chronic asthma and rhinitis due to Candida albicans, epidermophyton and trichophyton', *Annals of Allergy* 59 (1987): 48–51.

8. Ward *et al.*, 'Trichophyton asthma, reduction of specific bronchial hyper-reactivity following long-term anti-fungal therapy', *Journal of Allergy and Clinical Immunology* (Jan 1994).

9. Van Der Bremt, 'Ketoconazole in asthma. A pilot study', *Journal of Allergy and Clinical Immunology* (Jan 1994 [abstract]).

Chapter 9

1. *Science News* 133 (1988).
2. 'A synergism of antigen challenge and severe magnesium deficiency on blood and urinary histamine levels in rats', *Journal of the American College of Nutrition* 9.6 (1990): 616–22.
3. G. Rolla, 'Reduction of histamine induced bronchoconstriction by magnesium in asthmatic subjects', *Allergy* 42 (1987): 186–88.
4. Britton, 'Dietary magnesium, lung function, wheezing and airway hyper-reactivity in a random adult population sample', *Lancet* 344 (1994): 357–61.
5. 'The relation between magnesium, blood histamine level and eosinophilia in the acute stage of the allergic reaction in humans', *Arch Immunol Ther Exp* (WAR SZ) 26 (1–6; 1978): 709–12.
6. 'Intravenous magnesium sulphate for the treatment of acute asthma in the emergency department', *Journal of the American Medical Association* 262.9 (1989): 1210–13.
7. E. H. Brunner *et al.*, 'Effect of parentral magnesium on pulmonary function, plasma C-amp, and histamine in bronchial asthma', *Journal Asthma* 22 (1985): 3–11.
8. J. V. Wright, *JAQA* 1.4 (Feb 1988).
9. G. Bray, 'The hypochlorhydria of asthma in childhood', *Quarterly of Medicine* (Jan. 1931): 181–7.
10. S. W. Simon, 'Vitamin B_{12} therapy in asthma and chronic dermatoses', *Journal Allergy* 22 (1951): 183–85.
11. M. Caruselli *et al.*, abstracted in *Journal of the American Medical Association* 150.17 (1952): 1731.
12. Bray, *op cit.*
13. P. J. Collins *et al.*, 'Pyridoxine treatment of childhood bronchial asthma', *Ann Allergy* 35 (1975): 93–97.
14. Reynolds, 'Depressed plasma pyridoxine concentrations in adult asthmatics', *American Journal Clinical Nutrition* 41 (1985): 684–88.
15. Swartz, 'Dietary factors and their relation to respiratory symptoms. The 2nd National Health and Nutrition Examination Survey', *American Journal Epidemiology* 132.1 (1990): 67–76.
16. Mohsonin, 'Effect of vitamin C on NO_2 inducted airway hyper-responsiveness in normal subjects', *Amer Rev Respiratory Disease* 136 (1987): 1408–11.

17. Mohsonin, 'Effect of ascorbic acid on response to methacholine challenge in asthmatic patients', *Amer Rev Respiratory Disease* 127 (1983): 143–47.

18. C. O. Anah *et al.*, 'High-dose ascorbic acid in Nigerian asthmatics', *Tropical Geograph Med* 32 (1980): 132–37.

19. E. N. Schacter, 'The attenuation of exercise-induced bronchospasm by ascorbic acid', *Ann Allergy* 49.3 (1982): 146–51.

20. J. L. Malo, 'Lack of acute effects of ascorbic acid on spirometry and airway responsiveness to histamine in subjects with asthma', *Journal of Allergy and Clinical Immunology* 78.6 (1986): 32–58.

21. 'Treatment of childhood asthma with parentral vitamin B_{12}, gastric reacidification and the attention of food allergy, magnesium and pyridoxine. Three case reports with background and an integrated hypothesis', *Journal of Nutritional Medicine* 1 (1990): 277–82.

Chapter 14

1. J. R. Mansfield, B. J. Valler, M. J. Burrell and V. J. Curl, 'Treatment of equine allergic diseases with allergy neutralisation. A field study', *Journal of Nutritional and Environmental Medicine*.

2. J. B. Miller, 'A double-blind study of food extract in injection therapy', *Ann Allergy* 38.3 (1977).

3. W. J. Rea, 'Elimination of oral food challenge reactions by injection of food extracts', *Archives of Otolaryngology* 110 (1984): 248–52.

4. O'Shea, 'A double-blind study of children with hyperkinetic syndrome treated with multi-allergen extract sublingually', *Journal of Learning Disabilities* 14.4: 189–91.

5. Schiff, 'Broncho-provocation blocked by neutralisation therapy', *Journal of Allergy and Clinical Immunology* 71 (1983): 92.

6. J. Brostoff and G. Scadding, 'Low-dose sublingual therapy in patients with allergic rhinitis due to housedust mite', *Clin Allergy* 16 (1986): 483–91.

7. M. J. Radcliffe and J. Brostoff, 'Allergen-specific low-dose immunotherapy in perennial allergic rhinitis. A double-blind placebo-controlled cross-over study', *Journal of Investigational Allergology and Clin Immunology* 6.4 (1996).

8. R. Finn, 'A clinical trial of low-dose desensitization and environmental control', *Clinical Ecology* 4.2 (1988): 75–6.

9. D. S. King, 'Can allergic exposure provoke psychological symptoms? A double-blind test', *Biological Psychiatry* 16 (1981): 3–17.
10. C. W. Lehman, 'A double-blind study of sublingual provocative food testing', *Ann Allergy* 45 (1980): 144–49; D. L. Jewett, 'A double-blind study of symptom provocation to determine food sensitivity', *New England Journal of Medicine* 323 (1990): 429–33.
11. King *et al.*, 'Provocative neutralization. A 2-part study. Part 1 – The intracutaneous provocative food test. A multi-centre comparison study', *Journal of Otolaryngology* 9.3 (1988): 263–71.
12. King *et al.*, 'Provocative neutralization. A 2-part study. Part II – Subcutaneous neutralisation therapy. A multi-centre comparison study', *Journal of Otolaryngology* 9.9 (1988): 272–77.

Summary

1. *Quality in Healthcare* 1 (suppl. 2–8), 1992.

Index